Age Gracefully! New Science To Restore Your Mind and Body

Eliminate Senior Moments, Wrinkles and Low Energy!

Margianna Langston

HBS Strategies, Inc.
Decatur, GA 30033

Cover Design: Alek J., Upwork

Copyeditor and Formatter: Kim Carr, On the Mark Editorial Services

ISBN: 978-0-578-46165-6 (paperback)

ISBN: 978-0-9890575-0-9 (ebook)

This book is dedicated to my family and friends for their unwavering love and support at all times—the trouble-free and the challenging times. I also am grateful for the doctors, researchers, and other healthcare experts that have dedicated their work to searching "outside the box" to find solutions to major and prevalent healthcare problems and to improve preventive health.

Contents

Section One

~

Success Mindset and Goals

Introduction

Do you aspire to being a "senior cougar"? Hold on! Before you throw this book in the trash, let me describe my definition of a cougar and assure you that it is not the negative meaning that is in the dictionary. My senior cougar is a person with a beautiful and healthy body, a sharp and curious mind, and a peaceful soul!

So a senior cougar is not someone that flirts with younger men, flutters her eyelashes provocatively, wears low-cut tops, and acts like an immature twenty-year-old. **I am suggesting that she is someone that takes care of her spirit, mind, and body to achieve health, happiness and beauty.** Interested? Read on.

So what happens to your body as you age? Once you hit 40 years old, studies have shown that your body starts aging about six months extra for each additional year without the proper nutrients and exercise. **Steve and Becky Holman, editors of Iron Man Magazine,** report that by the time you hit 44, you will look and feel 48! And by the time you are 60, you will look and feel 70! Yikes! They say that 90 percent of people over the age of 35 lose enough muscle every year to burn off an additional four pounds of fat, so you not only lose shape, tone and strength but also gain fat each year. The Holmans go on to say that all this is reversible. "There are specific ways to move, eat, and think that tell your brain to STOP this rapid aging process ... or even SLOW IT DOWN to the point where you're aging less than a year for every year of age." That means you can look younger at 40 than you do at 35, or if you're like Steve and Becky, you look younger at 50+ than at 40!

You broadcast loud and clear that you are old if you are forgetful, have sagging skin, a wrinkled face, deep and dark circles under the eyes, crepey arms and legs, bad posture, yellow teeth, a weak voice, and a lack of energy and motivation. This book is for you if you want to reduce or eliminate these signs of old age and appear and feel more youthful and dynamic!

Herein, I'll divulge the secrets that keep movie stars and other celebrities and even ordinary people like us looking and feeling youthful. You'll also learn how your mind and spirit, as well as your body, control much of aging and anti-aging. The good news is I'll make it easy for you to achieve success—but only if you do your part and commit to doing what it takes.

**It's never too late to live the life you dreamed
(or have the mind and body that makes you happy)!!!**

Background

Let me tell you how and why I got interested in anti-aging. First of all, I have never been concerned about aging (even though I am now 81 years old) because I have always had abundant energy, good health, an active mind, a young look for my age, and a happy outlook. That is, until two years ago. Then, I had a debilitating (and dumb) thing happen to me. I was getting a very heavy glass mixing bowl off a high shelf, and it and four other glass bowls fell and hit me in the forehead. I was stunned and, thereafter, had a loss of balance and memory, dizziness, headaches, severe pain around my eyes and face, extreme fatigue, emotional stress, and blurred vision. I had suffered a concussion. Fortunately, after several weeks these symptoms subsided.

Two months later, I had cataract surgery on the eye below where I had the concussion and, incredibly, all my concussion symptoms immediately returned! The surgeon did not have an explanation for this nor did she accept any responsibility. I went to my primary care doctor, a neurologist, and two alternative care doctors and got some help but no significant improvements. My continuing symptoms unfortunately led to my body and mind perceptibly aging in the two years of having the post-concussion syndrome!

I was at a point where I had to accept an old age–like disability or accept that my happiness and health were up to me. This seemed almost overwhelming and, for sure, a big responsibility. However, even though I was somewhat skeptical but frustrated and at wit's end, I accepted the challenge. The long journey to find a cure began by relentlessly researching anti-aging and reversal of trauma to the brain and body. I was not only on a mission but also on a crusade!

Just recently, I learned a possible explanation of why I had a recurrence of concussion symptoms. **Dr. Norman Doidge, psychiatrist and psychoanalyst,** has spent decades researching traumatic brain injury and says that traumatic brain injuries need time to heal the inflammation and clear the toxins formed in the brain as a result of the injury; if that time for healing is not allowed, symptoms may continue and cause ongoing problems. Perhaps the cataract surgery caused further trauma to my brain. Maybe, maybe not!

It took a while, but I finally realized that my concussion occurred for a reason! Let me explain. I believe everything that happens in our lives is for a reason and a result of God's arrangements; events are not "good" or "bad." They are given to us to help us grow, to erase our negative karma, and/or to fulfill our life purposes . . . and ultimately improve our lives. I admit that my debilitating concussion symptoms were hard to think of as positive when I was hurting physically, mentally, and emotionally.

Finally accepting that something good would come from this, I shored myself up by offering service at my spiritual center, helping others, speaking positively to myself, and smiling.

Eventually, the good showed up. Hallelujah! As I found solutions to these difficult circumstances, I also gained the opportunity to fulfill my life's purpose: to help as many people as possible! This book fulfills my goal of showing retired adults how to feel valuable and useful and to be healthy!!!

Six months after the concussion (and I'm convinced as a result of the previous trauma to the brain), I had a mild stroke. In the two years since the concussion, followed by the stroke, I have tirelessly worked to overcome these symptoms even though my brain, body, and eyes haven't always cooperated and made it easy. I'm happy to report that I now function well enough to write and organize my writing; but, let me hasten to add that I won't stop my search to further repair my brain until it functions like a healthy 50-year-old's—a 60-year-old brain is not good enough!

Without this commitment to getting my brain and body back to normal, I could be severely handicapped by now. I discovered that the need is urgent for the old and young to follow healthy life practices to fully enjoy life into their senior years. Unfortunately, researchers now say that more and more young people, even those in their 30s and 40s, are experiencing dementia. But, this book is for those of us already in our senior years; however, younger people can also be helped. The following is what I have learned and, in many cases, practiced to give me back a sharp mind and healthy body.

Learn to thrive instead of just survive!

Choose to be Young

Recently, a woman at the gym aroused my curiosity, and I wanted to know more about her. Why? She is attractive, seemingly fit and, I thought, perhaps 60 years old. However, she seemed preoccupied with her exercise routine, so I didn't want to interrupt her. Consequently, I admired Jennifer from a distance as she worked out for about fifty minutes on a treadmill while reading a book.

One day, instead of exercising on the treadmill, she was riding a stationary bike, and I seized this time to speak to her. "I'm surprised to see you riding the bike instead of walking on the treadmill." She was friendly and said she thought that for best results, it was good to often change the type of workout.

We talked and I found out that she is also a writer and previously owned a company that specialized in advertising and public relations. After retiring, she began devoting her time to doing what she loves: using her artistic talent to paint pictures. And now her award-winning pastel art is shown in galleries and other businesses. I was impressed with her because she is clearly an interesting, energetic, intelligent, and talented woman.

Hesitantly, but out of genuine curiosity, I asked her how old she was. I was shocked when she answered "85 years old"! What?! It can't be; but then she had no reason to lie to me. I was curious to learn her secrets for staying young. It was obvious that several ingredients in maintaining her youth were exercising, having a purpose in life, and keeping her brain active. She shared with me that her faith, good diet, and supportive vitamins also play an important part in her health and happiness. Not surprisingly, each of these things is an important ingredient emphasized in the research for anti-aging. Jennifer intuitively has the answers for staying young and enjoying life!

But, you think. I am not Jennifer. I am 70 years old (or even only 60) and my face is sagging. I am depressed and have little energy. I'm overweight. I have senior moments. Now what?

Take heart! It's never too late and never too early!!!

Let's face it—nobody can go back and start over . . . but everyone can start today to make a new ending! It's still hard for me to admit that I'm 81 because I don't want to be treated like an old lady. Somehow, however, something happened when I hit 80; I was proud of my age, celebrated with a big party and enjoyed having people comment, "I can't believe you are 80." A 54-year-old friend commented on the many things we have in common for "our" age group. I responded, "I am closer to your 97-year-old mother's age than to yours." She said, "I think of you as a contemporary." Yes, me too!!!

The truth is, not much has changed since I was 50. I still have young friends and interests; entertain; visit my children and their families in Wyoming; love my Atlanta Falcons, Georgia Tech Yellow Jackets, and Atlanta United; and have a firm resolve that I have many more productive years ahead—with a sharp mind, healthy body, purposeful life, and attractive look!

Following is information that I hope you will enjoy that two of my friends posted about their mothers on my Facebook group page, *Life Starts After Forty:*

My friend's post: *This past weekend I realized I hadn't paid an insurance bill of my mother's that came due several weeks ago. For those who don't know, my mom is 90 and lives in a nursing home, but she still manages certain bills on her own and tells me what to pay. This year neither she nor I had seen the bill in question, so I tried calling the company this morning but was greeted with confusion. I finally learned from my mother that it was a cancer policy she had bought several decades ago, payable to her only if she needed treatment for cancer. She and I got on the phone with the company and, after jumping through hoops to trace it, I asked my mom outright if she really wanted to renew it. Her response was typical Mom: "Of course I want it. I'm getting to the age where I might need it!" Ninety years old!*

Another friend responded to the above Facebook post: *Reminds me of the time my siblings and I were able to get my mother into an assisted living facility. She was 88 years old. She greatly protested, saying, "But I don't want to be in there with all those old people!"*

Think Young to Be Young!

Listen up! Even at what has been considered "old age" in the past, you can be vivacious and create a fulfilling life. Depending on your condition, it may take a while, but you can be young in every way, that is, except for the actual number.

For the elderly or even newly retired . . . please consider: Have you given up? Do you feel your life is over? To be blunt, are you waiting to die? **Take heart—***it's never too late to choose to be valuable!* The question is how much do you want it? I can give you what is working for me in a step-by-step approach, but your commitment will be the determining factor in your remaining young and vital.

My goal is to help as many people as possible. But, as I have admitted, I learned what I did to regain my health and youthful appearance. With that said, not everyone has the passion or curiosity that I have for research and experimenting; therefore, I offer my service to others by sharing my knowledge.

I also confess that none of what I present in this book is original research or thinking. It comes from spending hundreds of hours and thousands of dollars on books and studying the experts as well as trial and error to determine what works. Think of me as your guinea pig with a thirst to find the answers. My goal is for all who are interested to have the information and tools they need to create an ageless spirit, mind, and body.

So, come with me on this exciting journey. We will deal with your subconscious mind first—that is, your beliefs and outlook, because nothing else will work if you are programmed inwardly for failure. With that dealt with, then we can move on to sharpen your brain (create and repair brain neurons), take away your wrinkles, create alluring eyes, skin, and hair, find glamorous clothes (and bargains) and, of utmost importance, help you find health and happiness. This book will conclude with everything you need to know in "Section Six: Recapture Your Youth" in a simple step-by-step eight-week plan. When you have accomplished this, send me a before and after picture! Don't forget, I'm here to virtually hold your hand all the way—you have a mentor!

As You Thinketh . . .

Do you believe that it is possible for you to be energetic and happy, and have a sharp mind and healthy body your entire life, even as a senior? Let me say up front that success will not come unless you believe it is possible!

Your body can stand almost anything. It's your mind that you must convince.

Keep reading, and in this chapter I'll give you the tools to make sure you have a supportive and positive mindset.

Frankly, you created an identity for yourself during childhood and reinforced this identity over the years with your thoughts and words. You have spent your life living up or down to the identity you've created for yourself. Often this identity has not come from what you consciously chose but from your childish and often misinterpreted observations; the actions and words of your parents, teachers, or other authority figures, as well as your own internal feelings. Unfortunately, as a child, your mind welcomes the input—good or bad—that surrounds you and possibly psychologically handicaps you.

To create a youthful and positive outlook as you grow older, you must believe that it can be a reality and that may mean changing who you think you are. The good news is that research now shows that we have the ability to change our internal (or childhood) programming and even our DNA!

Formerly, we believed we were stuck in a pattern, the one we created as a child. And it is true that to consciously change these ingrained beliefs may be next to impossible! To say "I love myself" or "I am worthwhile" or "I am beautiful" or other positive statements generally have little influence on our subconscious because our conscious mind blocks it. However, the good news is that there are techniques that bypass the conscious mind to change these negative beliefs. Scientists have proven that at any age, even as senior adults, there are ways we can change and replace the old, harmful programming with positive, productive programming.

So, if negative thoughts fill your mind that start with "I can't . . ." or "It's not possible . . ." or "I'm not . . ." and you want to create a new destiny for yourself, you have to commit to doing whatever it takes. First, literally wave goodbye to your old identity! Now, it will not be a cake walk. As I will say over and over again, your results will be proportional to your commitment. You have to be dedicated to changing and focused on carrying out this anti-aging and happiness program systematically and consistently.

COMMIT! COMMIT! COMMIT!

Your Subconscious Beliefs

Before you can change and achieve success in any endeavor, it is helpful (but not essential) to reflect and identify your belief system. You may think, "There is no way to know what is in my subconscious mind." Oh, yes, there is! All you have to do is look at your life and thoughts, and you can clearly see your unconscious beliefs.

For instance:

_____Do you think of yourself as young and vibrant, no matter or in spite of your age?

_____When you get out of bed, are you looking forward to the day?

_____Do you have purpose/goals in life for when you retire?

_____Are you healthy and energetic?

_____Are you happy with your life?

Congratulations if you answered "yes" to all of the above. However, you may be thinking, "You're kidding. That's a lot to ask of me." In many cases, we have limited ourselves all our lives. Some of us have been carrying around a burden of low self-esteem from our childhood when we were not appreciated or loved and possibly, even worse, told we were worthless.

Before we continue, let me put to bed the thought that your genes are controlling who you are. Research has now shown how little of our personality, behaviors, and internal psychological programming can be attributed to our genetics. Many people strongly believe that they are powerless to change because of their family history or their DNA. NOT TRUE!

From stem cell biologist Bruce Lipton, PhD: The DNA we are born with is not the sole determinant for our health and well-being.

Becoming Positive: Are You a Victim or Victor?

Several members of your family may have your same behavioral and physical characteristics, but it is likely from the family environment rather than genetic programming. Let go of the excuse that you can't change because "it runs in my family."

> Let me reiterate: *Your genes are not controlling who you are. Accept that you are in charge of your life. Excuses don't get you to your destiny.*

Are you ready to accept responsibility for yourself and your life? If so, read on. You are the only person in charge of your happiness.

Now, if you are not programmed for success, let's begin the journey to change by practicing the following exercises daily, without fail!

1. Ask an empowering question, write it on slip of paper, and post it somewhere in your home, car, desk, and other places where you will see it often.

   Examples:

   "Why am I youthful in body, mind, and spirit?"

   "Why am I healthy and wealthy?"

   "Why am I a perfect child of God?"

   Or you can choose another positive question. Repeat the question that you've posted over and over during the day.

   Noah St. John, author of Afformations, says to phrase affirmations as questions (afformations) and explains: "Because your brain's embedded presupposition factor, when you ask a question, either internally or externally, your brain is wired to search for the answer." [I did this exercise and wrote, "Why can I enjoy my wonderful wealth and still be spiritually centered?" Within two weeks, I received two unexpected checks.]

2. Gather together a memo pad, pen, and a container (such as a quart jar or a vase). Each night at bedtime, write in longhand a positive statement (or question) without lifting your hand off the paper. For example, "Why am I happy and

energetic?" or "Why do I have all the money I need to live comfortably?" Then trace the words with your fingers and place the paper in the container. Your dreams will then be programmed to push out the negative beliefs and embed the positive.

Dr. John Kappas, author of Success is Not an Accident: The Mental Bank Concept, *states that the subconscious mind is most receptive when a person is relaxed at bedtime, and when she writes a goal in longhand without taking her hand off the page, the thought is allowed to sink into the subconscious mind.*

3. Speak and think only positive words.

   "A man is but the product of his thoughts, what he thinks, he becomes."
   — Mahatma Gandhi

4. For one month, practice saying ***thank you*** many times every day, even when you are angry, hurt, sad, lonely, or feel life is dumping on you. Focus on your blessings NOW: what you have, what you are, and what you have been given. Be happy in the moment instead of "I'll be happy when …" and watch your life and thoughts change. Always be mindful that "this, too, will pass."

5. Imagery can be very powerful. By taking advantage of its power, you can successfully limit the number of negative thoughts that enter your mind. Picture yourself as you would like to become: how you would look, what you would say, and what you would think. (You are now the star of a movie based on the wonderful you!) The more you practice these images, the more likely you will see changes in your life!

   "In order to carry a positive action, we must develop a positive vision."
   — Dalai Lama

Gratitude Can Change Your Life

When I'm worried and I can't sleep,
I count my blessings instead of sheep
And I fall asleep counting my blessings

Since the song "Count Your Blessings" by Irving Berlin came out in 1954, many clinical studies have verified that gratitude is strongly related to aspects of well-being. So what does gratitude have to do with your outlook and brain health? Gratitude reduces stress, shortens recovery from illness, replaces negative thinking, and creates happiness; all of which help maintain your youth.

"Of all the attitudes we can acquire, surely the attitude of gratitude is the most important and by far the most life-changing."
— Zig Ziglar

Health, happiness, and prosperity are knocking on your door. Open that door with gratitude. Establish a habit of gratitude.

I, MARGIANNA, COUNT MY BLESSINGS ONE BY ONE . . .

I am grateful to live in the United States of America where I have freedom, safety, and peace.

Recently, I was visiting a friend who is paralyzed from the waist down. As background, here is her story:

Lee Hong: *Several years ago, a neurologist diagnosed my friend with Parkinson's disease and prescribed dopamine for her. After a couple years, the drug showed no signs of helping her symptoms, and her condition gradually worsened, causing leg disability. She then decided to get a second opinion and the new neurologist found she had been misdiagnosed, and, instead of Parkinson's, she actually had spinal stenosis that was causing her problems. The doctor operated two times without good results and said it was too dangerous to operate again. My friend became paralyzed below the waist.*

On a recent visit, we talked and she shared a story that has truly inspired me. She told me of watching PBS and seeing the story of the people in poverty in the many African countries. It showed graphic imagery of women holding their babies and young children who were so thin that their eyes bulged out and their bones protruded from their malnourished bodies. The mothers had no food to feed their children, and, with anguish, helplessly watched them die in their arms. My friend was disturbed by this, and so was I.

Then, my friend expressed gratitude that she lives in comfort, has food and many other conveniences, and is allowed to work from home. I was deeply affected by this story not only because of the plight of these starving families but also because my friend was expressing gratitude even though she has gone from a healthy, fully independent person to one who is paralyzed. She now requires a helper to get her in and out of bed morning and night—yet, she is grateful! What a wonderful example for us to follow.

I, Margianna, am grateful to be healthy and independent!

Eric Edwards, Your Abundance Coach: *"I actively practice gratitude. I firmly believe it to be the most powerful energy one can give to oneself and to The Universe."*

I, Margianna, am grateful to make a difference!

Oprah Winfrey: *"I live in the space of thankfulness—and I have been rewarded a million times over for it. Opportunities, relationships, even money flowed my way when I learned to be grateful no matter what happened in my life."*

Regional Director, Sukyo Mahikari North America *related that members at a center in Peru undertook reading the organization's book, Gratitude, at least nine times in order to understand the true significance of gratitude. Many lives changed, including those of nine people whose cancer disappeared.*

I, Margianna, am thankful to live in comfort, peace, freedom, and safety in the USA.

Aimee Copeland *is a 24-year-old West Georgia College graduate student who fell from a zip-line in May 2012 and contracted rare flesh-eating bacteria through a cut on her leg. Initially, she was clinging to life, on a respirator, and not expected to live. Eventually, her left leg, right foot, and both hands were amputated and a long rehabilitation followed. Aimee has inspired many with her positive attitude and zest for living and has never doubted that she would be independent again. She continued college and works to help disabled children. Recently, Aimee spoke to elementary school students, told them of her battle, and urged them to never give up on their dreams no matter how challenging. Aimee says her life is "full of blessings." Incredible!*

I, Margianna, thank God for my life!

Gratitude is an effective way to change your thinking and history from negative and destructive to positive and supportive. Even if you do not feel grateful, practice saying "thank you" or "I'm grateful for. . ." and remember your subconscious takes you at your word and does not judge whether you are being truthful or lying. Fake it until you make it! Practice until it becomes true.

**Gratitude can unlock your happiness—it is the key to a
happy and fulfilling life!**

Dedicate each day to inspiring many people by your example and by your positive encouragement and words. Help change this world!! We need you!

Gratitude Research

- Gratitude can reverse aging, stress, and illness: http://www.naturalnews.com/047287_gratitude_reverse_aging_stress.html

- The Healing Power of Gratitude: http://www.chopra.com/ccl/cultivate-the-healing-power-of-gratitude

- The new science of gratitude: http://gratitudepower.net/science.htm

Margianna's Tip

Before you get out of bed in the morning, express gratitude for having a good night's sleep, or if that is not the case, be grateful that you have a comfortable bed and home in which to sleep. Continue expressing gratitude as you go through the day for God's blessings (family, friends, food, clothing, creative ideas, healthy body, etc.).

* * *

Having practiced the steps in this chapter, do you now feel positive about rejuvenating your body, mind, and spirit? If not, commit to practicing and expressing gratitude daily until your outlook shifts. When you are feeling positive, continue reading and I will give you further steps that will lead to a youthful you.

Purpose in Life

Most people look forward to the age when they retire. The thought of relaxing, sleeping late, having more leisure time, and other positive activities is heavenly. My advice: **Don't do it. Don't retire!!** "But . . . but . . . but . . ." as you protest, "I've looked forward to retirement for many years. I've worked hard, I deserve this." Before you stop reading and/or think I've lost my (bleeping) mind, let me clarify. There is nothing wrong with retiring from your 9–5 job at 60, 65, 70 years old or younger! However, it is absolutely essential that you don't retire from life!

> **A goal or a purpose for living is necessary if you want to maintain a healthy brain and increase your longevity!**

In this chapter, I'll help you determine your purpose in life and show you how you can "make a difference" after retirement.

*Age hardly deterred **Annemarie Eaton of Atlanta**, my brother-in-law's mother. At 69, she put on a backpack, caught the bus, went to Georgia State University and earned a master's degree in gerontology (adding to the advanced degrees that were already hers). She wanted to help the "old people." Through the years, she wrote several books on aging that dealt with various subjects but carried a recurring theme: "Live a full life. Stay active." One granddaughter said, "She felt it was really important that, as people age, they stay intellectually, physically and socially engaged so that they can age gracefully."*

I can remember hearing that Anne wanted to move when she was 100 years old because she needed "a computer room!" I went to her 100th birthday party, attended by a ballroom of family, friends, and celebrities where Anne gave a talk about the value of education. She lived to be 102 years old, remaining active until the end in spite of having had a heart attack, stroke and cancer. She lived an inspiring life and will live on through the trust she set up for her great-grandchildren's college education.

It's never too late to live the life you imagined! Don't leave behind a wasted life!

I retired from my 9–5 job over 5 years ago . . . and now enjoy staying up until midnight, sleeping till 8 a.m. or later, leisurely styling my hair and putting on makeup while checking my email, Facebook, and watching TV, going to movies or lunch with friends and enjoying other daytime activities. The activities, however, that revitalize me and produce the most happiness are researching, writing, and offering service at my spiritual center! These activities are rewarding because they help me maintain a creative mind and carry out my purpose of helping others.

Many years ago, I asked a friend what she would do when she retired from teaching. I was appalled at her answer: "I'm going to lie on the couch and watch TV." After retirement, she did just that and, within a short period of time, she was disabled from an auto-immune disease. I can't say unequivocally that this wouldn't have happened if she had remained active carrying out a purpose, but, personally, I wonder.

Lead author Lei Yu from the Rush Memory and Aging Project told Reuters: *"We and others have shown that purpose in life is protective against multiple adverse health outcomes in older age . . . Importantly, purpose in life may be improved through changes in behaviors or participation in activities like* *volunteerism, among other things. . . Older people with a greater sense of purpose are less likely to develop adverse health outcomes, including decreased mortality, decline in physical function, frailty, disability, Alzheimer's disease, and clinical stroke."*

Don't sit on the sidelines of life!

Determine Your Purpose

What can you do? What will make you happy? Keep in mind as you determine your goals that challenging the brain will contribute to it remaining young and sharp. Being useful gives a sense of value. (By the way, setting goals and achieving them floods your brain with dopamine that gives a surge of pleasure.)

My purpose is _____.

Make a Difference

"But, I'm a small fish in a big pond." True, most of us think we are helpless to improve the world and people's lives. Forget that notion. YOU CAN MAKE A DIFFERENCE! How? By improving the life of even one person.

Random Acts of Kindness

Small acts of kindness can change the lives of friends and strangers and, ultimately, transform our world.

- *Several weeks ago, I was in my doctor's office, waiting to be called for my appointment. An elderly man and woman came in, both on walkers and*

21

helped by an attendant. After they were seated, the attendant left. The man then stood up while holding onto his walker to put on his sweater but couldn't get one arm in a sleeve. I thought, "Should I wait to see if he is successful, or should I help him?" After watching his struggles for several seconds, I decided to help. It took very little time and effort, but, nevertheless, the man was extremely grateful. (You would have thought I had given him the winning lottery ticket.) We began talking and he told me he and his wife lived at Wesley Woods, an Atlanta senior center, and really liked it there. Soon, the nurse called me to come in for my appointment, and as I walked in, the man said to the nurse, "You are taking away our good friend." This little "Random Act of Kindness" brightened this couple's day and put a long-lasting smile on my face.

- *A friend told me that when she is driving and sees a homeless person with a sign that includes "Need Food," she stops, gives him or her part of her lunch and $2.00. Often, we ignore these people, thinking they are frauds or taking advantage of us. But, what if they are not? My friend says it doesn't matter what their motives are; some truly need help and she can help.*

- *I recently read the following story on Facebook, posted by a local TV station: An 18-year-old works as a part-time greeter at Wal-Mart, and he noticed a man came in wearing no shoes, an oversized shirt, and oversized pants. Without hesitation, this young man took off his expensive pink Converse shoes and gave them to the man. Why? "I was homeless from age 8 until last year. When I was 13 and homeless, I complimented a man in my church on his shoes. He said, 'Do you want them?' Of course I wanted them and was thrilled." The young man continued, "Most people just don't understand what something so little can mean to somebody else in their life." The young man said his family has always instilled in him the value of a kind gesture, even when they had nothing.*

People need you and me!

A simple and effortless way to make a difference in people's lives is by saying kind words and offering support in small ways. Many people who are stressed and/or depressed have no one to encourage or love them and boost their spirits. The best way I can describe this is to relate the story of how one of my mother's friends inspired me to like myself.

- *When I was 11 years old, I felt very unattractive with a face full of freckles, a "large" nose, a pudgy body, unmanageable hair, and what I thought was a "blah" look. One day my mother's fashionable and attractive friend evidently sensed that I did not like myself and encouragingly said, "Margianna, when you get older and use a little bit of makeup, you are going to be very attractive!" Life changing! Yes, I hung on to those kind words during my insecure teen years.*

- *Many years ago, I was suffering. I was emotionally distraught, working for a tyrannical boss, etc., etc., etc. When I would feel very low and hopeless, I would call a friend to ask how she was doing. After talking with her without mentioning my situation, I forgot my distress, my spirits were lifted, and I was helped through many difficult days. By helping others, you help yourself.*

Hug your family and friends.

Hugging can have a therapeutic effect on the body and mind. The average length of a hug between two people is three seconds. But the researchers have discovered that when a hug lasts twenty seconds, a hormone called Oxytocin, known as the love hormone, is produced. This substance has many benefits in our physical and mental health; it helps us to relax, to feel safe and to calm our fears and anxiety. We give this wonderful gift free of charge every time we hold a person in our arms, cradle a child, cherish a dog or a cat, and/or dance with our partner. (I've told several friends the benefits of hugging, and so when we hug, they count down from twenty to one. When we finish hugging, we are both rejuvenated!)

Results of a hug, condensed from **Jen Reviews**, produced and authored by Jen Miller, award-winning freelance writer (contributor to the New York Times):

1. ***Stimulates Oxytocin*** — *Since hugging increases the body's capacity to release Oxytocin, hugging helps prevent aging.*

2. ***Cultivates Patience*** — *A hug is one of the easiest ways to show appreciation and acknowledgment of another person.*

3. ***Prevents Disease*** — *The Touch Research Institute at the University of Miami School of Medicine says it has carried out more than 100 studies on touch and found evidence of significant positive effects of hugging, including faster growth in premature babies, reduced pain, decreased autoimmune disease symptoms, lowered glucose levels in children with diabetes, and improved immune systems in people with cancer.*

4. ***Stimulates Thymus Gland*** — *Hugs strengthen the immune system.*

5. ***Communicates Without Saying a Word*** — *The interpretation of body language can be based on a single gesture, and hugging is an excellent method of expressing yourself nonverbally to another human being or animal.*

6. ***Self-Esteem*** — *Hugging boosts self-esteem, especially in children. Hugs, therefore, connect us to our ability to self-love.*

7. ***Stimulates Dopamine*** — *Hugs stimulate the brain to release dopamine, the pleasure hormone.*

8. ***Stimulates Serotonin*** — *Reaching out and hugging releases endorphins and serotonin into the blood vessels, and the released endorphins and serotonin cause pleasure, negate pain and sadness, decrease the chances of heart problems, help fight excess weight, and prolong life.*

9. ***Parasympathetic Balance*** — *Hugs balance out the nervous system.*

Hugging keeps you young and maintains muscle strength.

Volunteer

Researchers suggest that volunteering strengthens your sense of purpose and is a way to stimulate the prefrontal cortex, which analyzes, plans, and problem-solves. (And keeps your brain young.)

- *A Johns Hopkins study found that older women who tutored kids for six months developed sharper cognitive skills. The social and mental activity required for teaching sends blood rushing to the brain.*

- *When older adults volunteered in the Baltimore Experience Corps, a program in which retirees serve as mentors to children, age-related shrinking of the brain stopped, and some brains even grew slightly in size in the retirees, according to research from Johns Hopkins Bloomberg School of Public Health in Baltimore. (From AARP Bulletin, December 2017)*

Not only does volunteering impact the older volunteers but it has an incredible impact on the lives of the young. Older volunteers can use their wisdom and experience to revitalize their lives and make the world a better place.

Commit to something bigger than yourself!

What will you do today to make a difference and maintain a young brain?

Dr. Daniel Amen's Advice to College Graduates:

1. *Pray more about your path, relationships, and best ways to make a difference.*

2. *Always choose passion over money, if you have a way to support yourself.*

3. *Stop caring what others think of you and do the work God put you on Earth to do.*

Let's work together to change the world to a place of love, compassion, and happiness . . . one person at a time. What would heaven on earth be like? Let's find out. The next chapter will give you the techniques for achieving happiness.

Margianna's Tip

A famous quote by psychotherapist Virginia Satir goes, "We need four hugs a day for survival. We need eight hugs a day for maintenance. We need twelve hugs a day for growth." Whether those exact numbers have been scientifically proven remains to be seen, but there is a great deal of scientific evidence related to the importance of hugs and physical contact.

Happiness Is Your Choice

Happiness is a choice! Your happiness is not dependent on someone else or your circumstances, how you are treated, how much money you have, your health, or any other external thing. In this chapter, you will learn how to be happy (even when you are not).

Mark Rose says in his book ***Heaven on Earth***, *"You're probably coming up with exceptions such as, 'I can choose to be happy except when this happens, or I can choose to be happy as long as this person doesn't do that thing I don't like.'"*

It is not someone else that is undermining your happiness and success. You are doing it to yourself! You don't have to believe every stupid thought you have!

Only you are in charge of your happiness.

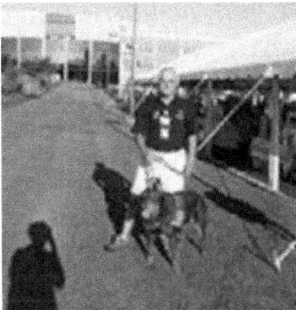

My brother-in-law has been a wonderful role model for me in choosing happiness. Goetz is a lovable character who thrives on interacting with and helping people. After retirement as Labor Relations Vice President of a Fortune 500 company, he took part-time jobs watering and selling plants at a popular big-box store and delivering hospital lab samples in his

South Carolina hometown. Although he had been a high-powered executive, he has enjoyed these jobs interacting with people and has never considered the jobs beneath his dignity or unimportant. When I visited him and my sister, I went to his store to get plants for my balcony garden. As we walked around the flower area, we were constantly interrupted by women who came specifically to talk to him and get his advice. He was gracious to all and always engaged the children in the women's carts (and gave them flowers). His wife, my sister, told me that this store in this small town had the largest sale of plants and flowers of any of the company's stores in the southeast, including Atlanta. She said that the store management credits the phenomenal success to Goetz.

But that's not all. After several years enjoying his part-time jobs, Goetz, at 79 years old (now 83), was asked to be a part-time judge for traffic and criminal cases in the Anderson Municipal Court.

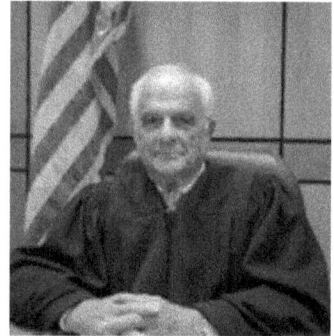

He has a history of working with the local courts mentoring young offenders and through the court, he has continued to help many young people who have gotten into trouble—while he also continues his work at the big-box store and the hospital.

You may dismiss Goetz's story because you think, "He's not like me. He has had an easy life, works for enjoyment, has no worries and loves what he does." Yes, he does work for enjoyment and doesn't need the money. But, he hasn't had a worry-free life. For years Goetz was under tremendous physical and emotional stress because of his wife's illness. Carolyn suffered through chemotherapy and radiation for over four years after receiving a cancer diagnosis. Goetz was her sole caretaker. Here is a "macho man" who never lifted a finger to help in their home who started cleaning the house, cooking meals, and grocery shopping. This was despite a poorly functioning heart as a result of three heart attacks. I have observed that he is often tired, but have never heard him complain or be negative. He goes out of his way to help and do things for people, including me. (I left the big-box store with my car's back seat full of flowers, for which Goetz insisted on paying.) Carolyn died several years ago, and Goetz was devastated; they met and had eyes only for each other since she was 15 years old and he was 16. Nevertheless, Goetz keeps his bright outlook, a smile on his face, and his focus on helping others. He inspires me. He is a wonderful example of a person who has taken charge of his own happiness! Thanks, GB!

OK, so Goetz is unusual. What if you don't feel like smiling? Maybe you are down in the dumps because you are lonely; owe a lot of money; your lover, husband, wife or friend has deserted you; or you are tired and sick. It doesn't matter!! You can change your mood in spite of your problems. How?

Fake it till you make it!

Smile

Smiling is contagious; it sends good vibes and can create positive change.

- *"Smiling can trick your brain into believing you're happy which can then spur feelings of happiness."* **Dr. Murray Grossan, a Los Angeles otolaryngologist,** *states that the study of the brain's connection with the immune system has shown "over and over again" that depression weakens the immune system while happiness strengthens the body's resistance. "When you smile, the brain sees the muscle activity and assumes that humor is happening."*

- **Dr. Isha Gupta, a neurologist from IGEA Brain and Spine** *explains that a smile (real or fake) "spurs a chemical reaction in the brain, releasing dopamine and serotonin." Dopamine increases our feelings of happiness.*

- ***Dr. David Perlmutter, neurologist and author***, *says to "consciously smile, for it will lower the level of cortisol [the stress hormone] in your body, so it is pretty dramatic."*

- ***Paul Ekman, PhD, a psychologist*** *who is an expert in facial expressions, taught himself to arrange the muscles in his face to make certain expressions. To his surprise, he found himself feeling the emotions that he was mimicking. Ekman and his research partner went on to do a study of college students to see if they, too, would feel happier when they followed instructions to smile using the muscles in their cheeks and around their mouths. The students' brain activity and happiness increased and was virtually the same whether their smile was genuine or fake.*

Neuro-linguistic Programming (NLP) teaches that external physiology—including posture and facial expression—can change internal emotions! Of course, this is opposite of the traditional belief that our moods are determined by our internal feelings.

Test the theory that by changing your physiology, you change your mood: Look into a mirror and stand with your shoulders back, chin up, and a smile on your face, then be depressed. Actually, you will find that it is impossible to be depressed if you maintain the suggested physiology.

Science has shown that the mere act of smiling can lift your mood, lower stress, boost your immune system, and maybe even prolong your life. Who wouldn't want to do this? Start incorporating a smile (and happiness) in your life!

As part of your morning routine, look in the mirror and smile for sixty seconds while adopting an upbeat physiology (shoulders back, spine straight, and chin up). This will begin your day with happiness and perhaps even lead you to happiness throughout the day.

> **EVERY TIME YOU SMILE AT SOMEONE, IT IS AN ACTION OF LOVE, A GIFT TO THAT PERSON, A BEAUTIFUL THING.**
> MOTHER TERESA

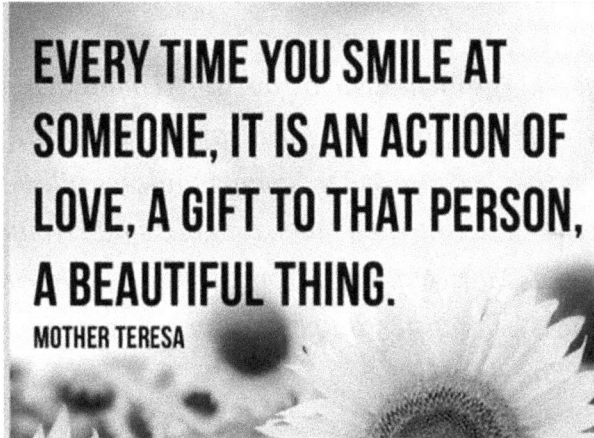

Smiling Experiences

My friend Annette's story as she tells it:

"One day when I smiled, Margianna told me how beautiful I looked when I smiled. She said that I should smile more often, and she would make it her responsibility to remind me by grinning at me every time she sees me. She also told me to look in a mirror and smile at myself. When I examined my face in the mirror, I was shocked to see that my mouth turned down and I looked unpleasant. Margianna later told me that prior to smiling, I always looked like I had lost my best friend!

"It is not an exaggeration to say that smiling has changed my life. I started smiling at everyone at work, something that wasn't easy for me in our impersonal government research environment. Eventually, my smiling in the office became contagious and resulted in a positive change in the demeanor of my coworkers. As I grinned at one co-worker, she remarked that I had beautiful teeth! I know that it wasn't my teeth but the smile that attracted her. I now feel positive energy is surrounding me and is affecting my family, friends, and coworkers. I've changed myself, and it changed my world!"

Maricela

Several times a week, I go to the gym to exercise. A couple of months ago, I noticed an employee there, a young woman who always looks pleasant and brightens my day each time I see her because of her glowing smile. I smile back and feel happy. We eventually began greeting each other, and this small, young Spanish woman introduced herself as Maricela. Before long, we started sharing small talk and I found out that she is helping her daughter plan her upcoming wedding, so she is not as young as I had thought.

Eventually, I asked Maricela if she liked her job at the Wellness Center, and smiling she replied, "Oh yes! I've been working here a year." I was tremendously impressed because, you see, her job is to clean the toilets, mop the floors, and keep the rest of the gym clean, and she does this always with a smile on her face. She is the housekeeper for the gym!

I wanted to be friends with Maricela and said to her, "I hope we can be friends someday." She replied with a big smile, "We are friends" and then she added, "You make me feel important!" I was moved to tears. She had it all wrong. It is Maricela that makes me feel important and brings happiness into my life as well as happiness into the lives of many other people. She does not realize the valuable lesson she has taught me in humility or the lesson of the importance of a smile.

Maricela is a perfect example of how we can influence others, as well as improve and change their lives by the simple act of smiling and sharing positive vibrations. (It also helps to practice humility.) We need more Maricelas to make a difference in this world. I'm grateful for these valuable lessons and will do my best to follow Maricela's example. Join Maricela and me in changing the world!

Smile and the world smiles with you!

Smile Exercise

- *Smile incessantly, at yourself and others. Make smiling and laughter a routine part of your day and life to improve your mood and add to the happiness of others.*

- *Smile when you are tense, such as when you're stuck in traffic, feel crummy, or even when you wake up with a headache.*

- *Smile and laugh yourself to health and happiness—you also are giving others a gift of joy.*

> **Be the reason someone smiles.**
> **Be the reason someone feels loved.**
> **When the world frowns, smile back.**

Laughter

Let's take the positive energy created with a smile one step further with laughter. Laughter is a powerful tool to heal the spirit, mind, and body! As in smiling, endorphins are released as we laugh, creating a feeling of euphoria and well-being. Laugh at all the silly problems you've been holding on to for so long. Laugh and be happy that you are alive and have many opportunities open to you—right now!

- *Mother: Anton, do you think I'm a bad mother?*
  Son: My name is Paul.

- *A nice old lady on a bus offers the driver some peanuts. He's happy to take some. He asks her after a while why she isn't having any herself.*
  "Oh, young man," she says, "they're too hard on my poor teeth, I couldn't."

"Why did you buy them at all then?" wonders the driver.
"You see, I just love the chocolate they're covered in!"

- *A woman was just taking a bath when she heard the doorbell. She thought she'd just pretend not to be home but then the ringer called, "Hello? Anybody home? I'm the blind guy!"*
"Ah well, if he is blind I can go and open the door just like this. No need to dress," thought the lady who then hauled herself out of the bath and went to open the door.
"Wow," said the guy waiting there, "you should be on a fitness studio advertisement! Now, where should I put these blinds?"

- *Yesterday I wore something from ten years ago and it fit!!! So proud of myself. It was a scarf. OK . . . Let's be positive.*

- *Research has shown that people eat more bananas than monkeys. I believe that . . . because I have never eaten a monkey!*

You are on your way to health and happiness if you laughed at the above humor!

Benefits of Laughter

The Spirit

- Creates an optimistic outlook through difficult times and suffering
- Diffuses conflict
- Heals relationships and unites people
- Promotes joy

The Mind

- Eases anxiety and fear
- Relieves stress
- Improves mood

The Body

- Boosts immune system
- Decreases or eliminates pain
- Relaxes muscles
- Improves heart health

Laughter Exercise

- Look in the mirror and fake a laugh (ha, ha, ha). I find that after doing this for several seconds I start literally laughing at myself.

Other Happiness Activities

Sing!

Singing for ten minutes a day:

- Increases happiness
- Relieves pain
- Reduces stress
- Increases longevity
- Clears sinuses

Release Oxytocin

There are many ways to consciously release the happiness/love hormone to increase your well-being, reduce stress, and live longer and healthier. Oxytocin, the happiness neurotransmitter, is produced in the brain by the hypothalamus by:

- *Giving money away – showing compassion is connected with higher levels of Oxytocin.*

- *Hugging – touching and hugging releases Oxytocin, especially in a prolonged hug of at least twenty seconds. Almost as good as hugging is imagining yourself being hugged by someone you love. (The brain works in remarkable ways!)*

- *Facebook – Like a post by a random friend. It releases Oxytocin. Who knew?*

- *Watch comedies (movie or TV), laugh and experience your Oxytocin catching fire!*

- *Walking – meet with a friend to walk: have fun, enjoy an adventure, and feel thrilled.*

- *Phone calls – call friends and family and vocally hug people today.*

- *Speak positive words and think positive thoughts - your subconscious will respond and be positively reprogrammed.*

- *Music – listening to soothing music releases Oxytocin.*

- *Food – eggs, bananas and peppers are known to release Oxytocin.*

- *Breathing – deep breathing tricks your body into thinking everything is calm. When your body is calm, so is your mind.*

Ways to create happiness in the face of negativity:

- *Do not respond when a person is unpleasant or says negative things about you.*

- *Take every opportunity to say something positive to the person that has been unpleasant to you.*

- *Watch with interest and delight as the relationship changes.*

Happiness is a choice. Take charge of your happiness!!!

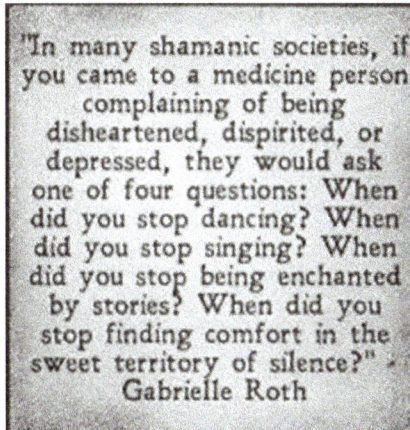

"In many shamanic societies, if you came to a medicine person complaining of being disheartened, dispirited, or depressed, they would ask one of four questions: When did you stop dancing? When did you stop singing? When did you stop being enchanted by stories? When did you stop finding comfort in the sweet territory of silence?" - Gabrielle Roth

Now that you are happy, read on to learn how to regenerate and repair your brain.

Section Two

~

It's All in Your Head – Regenerate and Repair Your Brain Cells

Previously, we discussed determining your subconscious beliefs while changing the negative ones and determining your purpose after retirement. These are all important but are negated when your brain is not functioning efficiently or properly or, heaven forbid, you have "senior moments."

"I hold that the brain is the most powerful organ in the human body."
— Hippocrates

So, the next important step is to create or maintain a healthy brain; that is, a healthy neural network. There are many ways to improve your brain function that will be discussed in this chapter and the following sections.

*Max Lugavere, author of **Genius Foods**, says that "your brain is capable of storing nearly eight thousand iPhones' worth of information. Everything you are, you do, love, feel, care for, long for, and aspire to is enabled by an incredibly complex, invisible symphony of neurological processes."*

Our society participates in systematically ravaging our brains with toxic and nutrient devoid foods, stress, lack of sleep, and medications, as well as many other ways. According to the Alzheimer's Association, an estimated 5.7 million Americans of all ages are living with Alzheimer's dementia in 2018. This number includes an estimated 5.5 million people age 65 and older and approximately 200,000 individuals under age 65 who have younger-onset dementia.

How do we change these statistics and eliminate the risks factors? Research has proven that a healthy brain will result from adopting a healthy lifestyle. New alternative therapies also show promise for the ability to create or regain a young, functioning brain into a person's senior years.

*From **Emory University's Biohacking Your Brain's Health Course**: "The brain is very plastic. Just like a muscle, the more you use the muscle, the bigger it gets. If you don't use it, you lose the bulk of that muscle, same thing happens in the brain."*

__Miia Kivipelto, a neurobiologist at Stockholm's Karolinska Institute__, is a foremost researcher exploring the effects of diet and lifestyle on the brain. The success of a trial he conducted highlights the power that a full lifestyle "makeover" can have on dramatically improving the way your brain works, even in old age.

Cognitive decline is not an inevitable part of aging!!!

The first step is to understand the latest research on "neurogenesis." Neurogenesis is how the brain renews and upgrades itself, the process of creating new brain cells (neurons). Over the years, the common belief has been that brain cells die as we get older and that's why we age—that is, until recently. The brain is now considered to be resilient, pliable, and plastic. Just like the muscles of the body, when the brain is well-nourished and stimulated through proper exercise, it heals and grows. And with proper care and feeding, this amazing brain regeneration can occur throughout life.

Breakthroughs have occurred in the last few years that have revolutionized how we perceive brain function. Some of these breakthroughs follow:

- The brain continues growing new brain cells during a person's entire life— lifelong neuroplasticity (the ability of the brain to change up until death) is possible.

- The rate of creating new brain cells varies greatly from person to person.

- Quality of life is important. An enriched environment can increase the rate of neurogenesis by three to five times at all ages, including in the elderly.

- At any age, seniors can be smarter, have a better memory, and be more vibrant, happy, and resistant to stress.

*Dr. Brant Cortright, a specialist in cutting-edge brain health and neuroscience therapy, details specific ways to prevent cognitive decline, dementia, and Alzheimer's in his book **The Neurogenesis Diet & Lifestyle: Upgrade Your Brain, Upgrade Your Life**. He is convinced that brain enhancement equals life enhancement.*

__Dr. Daniel Amen__, double board-certified Psychiatrist, Professor and Brain Health Expert, promotes "learn[ing] something new at least 15 minutes a day to exercise your brain."

Stop learning and your brain starts dying!

Following is a list of ways to regenerate brain cells that world experts gave in an interview by Peggy Sarlin in the webinar series **Awakening from Alzheimer's** and **Regain Your Brain** and by Dr. Cortright in his book **The Neurogenesis Diet & Lifestyle: Upgrade Your Brain, Upgrade Your Life**:

- Diet

- Physical Exercise

- Brain Exercises

- Supplements

- Sleep
- Social Network
- Spiritual Connection

Sayer Ji, founder of **Greenmedinfo.com** and vice chairman of the board of the National Health Federation, suggests the following to regenerate brain cells:

- Get lots of physical exercise
- Use stress reduction techniques
- Take strategic supplements
- Eat your veggies
- Employ continuous learning

Dr. Dale Bredesen, Founding President and CEO of the Buck Institute for Research on Aging, states that "Alzheimer's should be rare." He also believes that we're at the dawn of the era of treatable Alzheimer's.

In some cases, the experts relate case histories of severe dementia and debilitating Alzheimer's being totally reversed using the non-traditional methods described in the following sections. Review the information on each of the factors that impact brain neurogenesis and decide what you are willing to do to have a healthy brain . . . forever!

Diet

You have the option of being healthy or unhealthy: eat nourishing food or eat junk food! It's simple but not easy. You can choose to stay young and healthy in body and mind (or not) by your food choices. In this chapter, you will learn how to eat for your brain and body's health.

As a rule, the experts recommend a diet high in "good" fats, moderate in protein, low in carbohydrates, and devoid of processed and refined foods that result in inflammation in the body. I also learned many years ago that "systematic undereating" is the key to a long life.

> **Dr. David Perlmutter,** *neurologist and recipient of the prestigious Linus Pauling Award, says that the "food you eat can determine your genetic destiny. Your genes are turned on or your genes are turned off with every bite you eat" and adds that much of what we are advised to eat is "downright dangerous." He believes that more than 70 percent of our DNA that determines our health and longevity is directly affected by our lifestyle choices, predominantly our food choices. He believes that being overweight is a major cause of poor health and says, "The bigger your belly, the greater your risk for disease."*

The Amen Clinic:

High-fructose corn syrup is deadly to the brain and hormones. The Amen Clinic reports a study conducted at the University of California, Los Angeles, where researchers fed two groups of rats a solution containing high-fructose corn syrup—a common ingredient in processed foods—as drinking water for six weeks and, additionally, fed one group DHA supplements. Those who were not fed DHA supplements had developed signs of resistance to insulin, a hormone that controls blood sugar and regulates brain function.

Everyone is always focused on the effects of high-fructose corn syrup on weight gain and obesity, but this study shows that a high-fructose diet not only harms the body but also harms the brain.

High-fructose corn syrup is commonly found in soda, condiments, applesauce, baby food, and other processed snacks. What is worse is that the average American consumes more than forty pounds (18 kilograms) of high-fructose corn syrup per year according to the US Department of Agriculture.

The Standard American Diet (SAD)

The Standard American Diet (SAD) is saturated with sugar, high omega-6 fatty acids, excessive calories, trans fats, and processed and pesticide-laden foods. People who have a simple, carbohydrate-based diet (bread, pasta, potatoes, rice, fruit juice and sugar) have a 400% increased risk of getting Alzheimer's disease. New research has also linked a sugar-laden diet to diabetes and some scientists are now calling Alzheimer's "type 3 diabetes."

> The **standard American diet** leads to **standard American diseases** that lead to **standard American deaths.**

Alzheimer's disease, diabetes, depression, and obesity are national health epidemics that continue to grow. The answer is NOT to see them as individual, separate disorders but rather as different outcomes of the same unhealthy lifestyle that have exactly the same cure. The best way to prevent Alzheimer's is to eliminate all the risk factors that are associated with the disease—and the good news is that most of them are easily removed from one's life.

> Have I scared you enough or, better still, inspired you sufficiently that you will now eat to nourish your brain and prevent disease?

The "Dirty Dozen" Always buy these fruits and vegetables grown organically because they top the list of foods with the highest levels of pesticide residues:

- strawberries
- spinach
- nectarines
- apples
- grapes
- peaches
- cherries
- pears
- tomatoes
- celery
- potatoes
- sweet bell peppers
- hot peppers

Also avoid processed foods; that includes, those without fiber, refined, or packaged, and have a long lists of ingredients. They not only fail to promote good health but actually promote illness. Remember, a lot of what is sold in the grocery store is processed junk and is neither whole nor food.

The "Clean Fifteen" Fruits and vegetables grown with the least pesticide residue:

- avocado
- sweet corn – non-GMO
- pineapple
- cabbage
- onion
- sweet peas, frozen
- papaya
- asparagus
- mango
- honeydew melon
- kiwi
- cantaloupe
- cauliflower
- broccoli

Fermented foods contribute good bacteria that create a protective lining in the intestines that can improve digestion, boost immunity, help heal the gut, promote a healthy weight, and more. Sauerkraut, made from cabbage, and kimchi, made from Chinese cabbage and vegetables including cucumbers, ginseng and garlic, contain live microorganisms. Benefits of sauerkraut include its ability to enhance digestive health, reduce inflammation, stimulate the immune system, increase blood circulation, protect heart health, provide energy, strengthen bones, reduce overall cholesterol levels, protect against certain cancers, and even improve vision and skin health.

Kefir, kombucha, and apple cider vinegar are also beneficial fermented products while carrots, beets, kale, collards and celery spiced with ginger and garlic can also be fermented. Buy organic, raw and unfiltered veggies to ensure you are getting good quality produce.

Foods That Nourish Brain Cells

Dr. Brant Cortright, author of **The Neurogenesis Diet & Lifestyle: Upgrade Your Brain, Upgrade Your Life**, lists the following foods that maintain and/or create healthy brain cells:

1. *Blueberries*

2. *Green tea*

3. *Ginger*

4. *Curcumin, found in the spice turmeric*

5. *Whole soy foods such as tofu [Note: other experts do not recommend eating soy foods because of their influence on hormones]*

6. *Healthy fats*

    a. *Olive oil*

    b. *Avocados*

    c. *Coconut oil*

    d. *Fish or krill oil*

    e. *Flax oil*

7. *Raw nuts*

8. *Eggs*

9. *Pasture-raised butter*

Sayer Ji, Founder, GreenMedInfo LLC, recommends *Eat Your Veggies* – Stimulate brain cell regrowth by adding some freshly steamed broccoli to your meal. Science has added a substance called sulforaphane, found in sulfur-rich vegetables such as broccoli that is documented to stimulate nerve growth in the brain.

Foods and Behaviors That Destroy Brain Cells

1. *Overeating – obesity and diabetes are leading causes of dementia.*

2. *Sugar – provokes chronic inflammation. Eliminate all sources possible (except the sugar in natural foods like fruit), including table sugar, brown sugar, raw sugar, maple, rice and sorghum syrup, molasses, corn sweetener, dextrose, fructose, glucose, barley malt and concentrated fruit juice.*

3. *Excess of oils high in omega-6 – polyunsaturated vegetable oils like sunflower, corn, safflower, cottonseed, and grape seed oils are high in omega-6 and low in omega-3, and this contributes to premature aging and disease.*

4. *Grain-fed meat, eggs, and dairy – animals are fed diets of corn and soy, not their natural foods, in order to rapidly and excessively fatten them up. The result is sick animals, so they are injected with antibiotics and also hormones to fatten them up further.*

5. *Hydrogenated fats/trans fats – these are artificial fats that promote inflammation, insulin resistance, high cholesterol, and obesity. They are prevalent in deep-fried foods, commercial baked goods, and fast foods. Also, margarine, vegetable shortening, and partially hydrogenated oil are loaded with trans fats and should be avoided.*

6. *Caffeine – excessive ingestion of caffeine.*

7. *Alcohol – a healthy person can consume a glass of red wine or beer daily and receive health benefits. When more than these moderate levels of alcoholic*

beverages are consumed, inflammation is provoked, especially in the liver and esophagus.

8. *Processed foods – included are refined grains, processed meat, and pasteurized dairy. Refined grains have their nutritional value stripped; processed meat is a strong contributor to aging and disease, especially cancer of the colon and rectum and; pasteurization kills off the digestive enzymes.*

9. *Artificial ingredients - aspartame, saccharin, BHA and BHT, mono-sodium glutamate, sodium nitrate, and nitrite are artificial and not meant to go into the body! Many have been linked to serious diseases, including cancer.*

> If you want to look younger, feel younger, heal and prevent disease, and live longer, eat whole and natural foods and avoid foods with artificial ingredients.

***Eat This, Not That* by David Zinczenko** for staying young, weight loss and health [Note: Some of the tips are great advice; some are not recommended by other experts, including drinking milk* and eating wheat or rye.*]

1. *Drink a second cup of coffee. It might lower your risk of adult-onset diabetes, according to a study in the American Journal of Clinical Nutrition.*

2. *Keep serving dishes off the table. Researchers have found that when people are served individual plates, as opposed to empty plates with a platter of food in the middle of the table, they eat up to 35 percent less!*

3. *Think before you drink. The average person drinks more than 400 calories a day—double what he or she used to—and alone gets around ten teaspoons of added sugar every single day from soft drinks. Swap out sweetened teas and sodas for no-cal drinks and you could lose up to 40 pounds in a single year!*

4. *Practice total recall. British scientists found that people who thought about their last meal before snacking ate 30 percent fewer calories that those who didn't stop to think. The theory: Remembering what you had for lunch might remind you of how satiating the food was, which then makes you less likely to binge on your afternoon snack.*

5. *Eat protein at every meal. Dieters who eat the most protein tend to lose more weight while feeling less deprived than those who eat the least protein. It appears that protein is the best nutrient for jumpstarting your metabolism, squashing your appetite, and helping you eat less at subsequent meals.*

6. **Choose whole-grain bread. Eating whole grains (versus refined-grain or white bread) has been linked to lower risks of cancer and heart disease.*

   [Note: Two slices of whole wheat toast can create an unhealthy spike in blood sugar and high blood sugar over time makes you gain weight and age faster.]

7. *Think fish. Consuming two 4–6 ounce servings of oily fish a week will sharpen your mind. Among the best: salmon, tuna, herring, mackerel, and trout.*

8. *Sign up for weight-loss e-mails. Daily e-mails (or tweets) that contain weight-loss advice remind you of your goals and help you drop pounds, researchers from Canada found.*

9. *Cut portions by a quarter. Pennsylvania State University researchers discovered that by simply reducing meal portions 25 percent, people ate 10 percent fewer calories—without feeling any hungrier.*

10. *Turn off the TV. Scientists at the University of Massachusetts found that people who watch TV during a meal consume, on average, 288 more calories than those who don't eat with the tube on.*

11. *Put your fork down when you chew. Or take a sip of water between each bite—eating slowly can boost levels of two hormones that make you feel fuller, according to Greek researchers.*

12. **Choose rye (not wheat) bread for breakfast toast. Swedish researchers found that rye eaters were fuller 8 hours after breakfast than wheat-bread eaters, thanks to rye's high fiber content and minimal effect on blood sugar.*

13. *Eat a handful of fruit and vegetables a day. In one study, people who ate four or five servings scored higher on cognitive tests than those who consumed less than one serving.*

14. *Sip green tea. It might help you build a strong skeleton, say researchers in China, and help protect you from broken bones when you're older.*

15. *Work out before lunch or dinner. Doing so will make the meals you eat right afterward more filling, according to British researchers—meaning you'll eat fewer calories throughout the day.*

16. *Hung over? Choose asparagus. When South Korean researchers exposed a group of human liver cells to asparagus extract, it suppressed free radicals and more than doubled the activity of two enzymes that metabolize alcohol.*

17. *Sleep 8 hours a night. Too much or too little shut-eye can add extra pounds, say Wake Forest University researchers.*

18. *Discover miso soup. Brown wakame seaweed (used in miso soup) can help lower your blood pressure, especially if your levels are already high, say researchers at the University of North Carolina.*

19. **Drink two glasses of milk daily. People who drink the most milk have about a 16 percent lower risk of heart disease than people who drink the least.*

20. *Take a zinc supplement. It will motivate your immune cells to produce more of a protein that fights off bacterial infections.*

Feel-Good Foods

1. *Foods high in omega-3 have been scientifically proven to reduce depression and increase happiness. These foods include oily fish such as salmon, nuts, and flax seeds.*

2. *Foods rich in tryptophan, which is converted by the body into feel-good chemical serotonin. Lobster, turkey, pineapple, tofu, and bananas are high in tryptophan.*

3. *Foods with lots of amino acids that balance your mind include chicken, turkey, fish, cheese, cottage cheese, eggs, milk, nuts, bananas, avocados, and legumes.*

4. *Foods that raise Vitamin B levels that help safeguard against depression include spinach, peas, orange juice, and avocado.*

Dr. Axe describes "superfoods" as natural, nutrient-dense compounds that contain high concentrations of essential nutrients with proven health benefits. They're high in vitamins, minerals, omega-3 fatty acids, probiotics, or antioxidants … just to name a few!

Superfoods for Anti-Aging [Note: Dr. Axe also has different superfoods lists for weight loss and muscle building in his e-book.]

1. *Wild Salmon — Fish has a reputation of being a "brain food." Plan to eat a seafood meal four days a week, including salmon at least two times a week. Salmon is an excellent source of astaxanthin and omega-3 fatty acids that slow the effects of aging, both inside and outside the skin.*

   - *Reduces oxidative stress and inflammation, and enhances the immune system*

   - *Relieves arthritis*

- *Protects heart from disease*

- *Reduces the risk of a debilitating stroke*

- *Improves blood lipids*

- *Promotes healthy blood vessels*

- *Reduces mental disorders, including Alzheimer's*

2. *Avocado — Helps the body absorb other fat-soluble nutrients as well.*

- *One slice with a meal helps the body digest nutrients in other foods*

- *Naturally balances hormones with high levels of omega-9 fats*

- *Hydrates skin*

- *Reduces risk of cardiovascular disease*

- *Reduces inflammation*

- *Increases good HDL cholesterol levels*

- *Protects cells from damaging free radicals*

- *Contains carotenoids which provide vitamin A for eye health, boost the immune system, and support a healthy reproductive system.*

An avocado a day keeps aging away!

3. *Garlic — Antibacterial, antimicrobial, anti-inflammatory, anti-coagulant, antiseptic, and anti-fungal.*

- *Slows down the aging process*

- *Protects against pollutants and fights off toxins that can harm the immune system*

- *Has the power to kill dangerous viruses, bacteria, parasites, and cancer cells, according to the University of Maryland Medical Center.*

4. *Blueberries — Organically grown and wild blueberries have significantly higher concentrations of antioxidants than commercially grown fruit and provide more benefits when eaten raw.*

5. *Raspberries — similarly high in antioxidants to blueberries.*

   - *Support healthy skin and gums*

   - *Fight cancer cell growth*

   - *Reduce inflammation*

   - *Improve memory*

   - *Fight risk of Alzheimer's*

6. *Cocoa — main ingredient of dark chocolate and is high in antioxidants.*

   - *Enhances the mood*

   - *Protects the skin from UV sun damage*

   - *Boosts cardiovascular health and keeps arteries clear*

   - *Beneficial for the nervous system*

   - *Helps lower blood pressure*

   - *Reduces blood clots*

   - *Improves the skin*

   - *Sharpens the mind*

   - *Slows down the signs of aging*

7. *Indian Gooseberries (amla) — good source of dietary fiber, vitamin C, and minerals with great antioxidant properties which help slow the aging process. Gooseberries' benefits:*

   - *Increase red blood cell production*

- *Push out toxins, strengthen heart muscles and are beneficial to diabetics as they reduce blood sugar*

- *Good for skin, hair, and eyes*

- *Help balance stomach acids*

Jack LaLanne was a chiropractor, nutrition expert, and fitness trainer. At age 66, he tied ten boats around his waist that were carrying seventy-seven people, swam and pulled the boats one mile in less than one hour. . . . Incredibly, he performed a similar feat again at age 95! How'd Jack do it? His number one rule for nutrition was, "If man made it, don't eat it." Jack aged significantly slower than most people because he ate healthily and exercised daily.

Margianna's Tip

The main thing to remember about the food you eat to stay young is eat natural foods and avoid processed foods and foods loaded with chemicals. If you stick with organic meat, fish, and chicken, vegetables and low-carb fruit, you will not only be healthier but also lose weight, look younger, and maintain mental sharpness.

Exercise

> *Me:* Sobbing my heart out, eyes swollen, nose red . . .
> "I can't see you anymore . . . I am not going to let
> you hurt me like this again!"
>
> *Trainer:* "It was a sit-up. You did only one sit-up."

OK, I understand if exercise is not something you enjoy doing. I admit that I don't look forward to exercising; however, I am serious about and committed to keeping a sharp mind and healthy (and good-looking) body. Therefore, whether I feel like it or not, I force myself to go to the gym three times a week. [Let me note that most seniors on Medicare can get an insurance plan that provides SilverSneakers, a free gym membership.]

If you don't like to exercise, it doesn't matter; do it anyway—but only if you want to stay young and attractive in body and healthy in mind. Choose from the following exercises to maintain or regain a young look and sharp, well-functioning mind.

No matter your age, the best exercise for you is the one you enjoy the most and that is beneficial. As you decide what is best for you, it is important to keep in mind what you need to get out of your workout.

Dr. Barbara Bergin, an orthopedic surgeon in Austin, TX

For older adults, the number one priority must be maintaining your quality of life outside the gym. Dr. Bergin says to do that, focus on workouts designed to help you build strength, maintain muscle mass, stay mobile, and improve balance and stability.

> **Consult your doctor before starting any type of exercise to get advice concerning its safety for your condition and health.**

Before I relate the experts' opinions on exercise, I want to caution that many diverse and opposing points of view and exercises are included below. Each has value to certain people. Review the following and present those that you would enjoy and that you think would be beneficial to your health to your healthcare provider for approval.

Aerobic Exercise

Can sweating make you smarter? Yes, if you are sweating because of aerobic exercise. Scientists have discovered that exercise is good for the brain including improving memory, concentration, and abstract reasoning among older adults and may delay the onset of Alzheimer's.

Exercise Your Brain, AARP Magazine, March & April 2008: Waneen Spirduso, Ed.D, Professor at University of Texas at Austin and author of Exercise and Mediating Effects on Cognition

Aerobic exercise increases blood flow to the brain that nourishes brain cells and allows them to function more effectively. Dr. Spirduso says "exercise is kind of like making sure your engine is all tuned up. You can get cognitive benefits with activity that is fairly simple, like walking twenty minutes a day."

Many times brain fog comes with age, and exercise changes the brain to eliminate this and protect memory and thinking skills.

University of British Columbia

Researchers found that regular aerobic exercise, the kind that gets your heart and your sweat glands pumping, appears to boost the size of the hippocampus, the brain area involved in verbal memory and learning. Resistance training, balance, and muscle toning exercises do not have the same results, although they are important and provide other benefits to health.

The direct benefits of exercise come from its ability to reduce insulin resistance, reduce inflammation, and stimulate the release of growth factors. Indirectly, exercise improves mood and sleep and reduces stress and anxiety. Problems in these areas frequently cause or contribute to cognitive impairment.

Craig Castanet, D.C., CEDIR, CFMP, Backstrong Non-Surgical Rehab Clinic, Decompression Therapy, Decatur, GA (http://backstrong.net/)

Dr. Castanet is one of my very knowledgeable doctors, and I asked him to write about what he thought was the best exercise to maintain a healthy and attractive body. Following is his opinion:

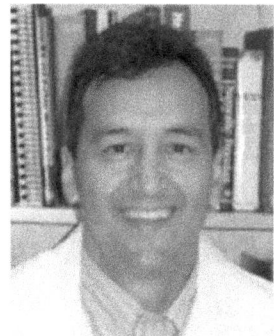

What is the best exercise? Exercise is the contraction of skeletal muscle(s). The best exercise is that which contracts all the major skeletal muscles, providing an anabolic stimulus. There is only one 'exercise' that works all the major skeletal muscles—that is, one exercise whose OBJECTIVE is to work all the major skeletal

muscles, and provide the anabolic stimulus that makes an organism superior in all bodily systems. That exercise is weight training.

Weight training is actually many exercises. Most other 'exercise' is better described as activity. Analyze all activity/exercises by deconstructing the various parameters of exercise, i.e., the muscles involved, the range of motion involved, the number of motor units recruited, and the number of repetitions. Critically analyzed, it is apparent that weight training is the best exercise. Weight training is also the reason that athletes are superior today than yesteryear.

In my personal and professional experience, weight training is the most potent means of improving one's strength, function, body composition, mood, libido, and mental health. And weight training is proven to improve all eleven of the body's systems—skin, muscular, skeletal, nervous, circulatory, lymphatic, respiratory, hormone, urinary, reproductive, and digestive.

Sarcopenia

Resistance training [weight training] is recommended to reverse or prevent Sarcopenia, an age-related condition that leads to the loss of skeletal muscle mass and strength. (https://healthyinfodaily.com/7-symptoms-of-sarcopenia; https://en.wikipedia.org/wiki/List_of_weight_training_exercises)

University of Illinois postdoctoral researcher Agnieszka Burzynska and director Art Kramer of Beckman Institute for Advanced Science and Technology Study:

"We looked at 100 adults between the ages of 60 and 80, and we used accelerometers to objectively measure their physical activity over a week." Their study suggests that more-fit older adults are more flexible, both cognitively and in terms of brain function, than their less-fit peers.

Balance

The Centers for Disease Control and Prevention

Stay out of the ER by improving your balance! The CDC reports that 7.8 million older adults visit the emergency room each year because of falls and more than 800,000 are hospitalized because of injuries from falls.

Donna Eden, author of The Eden Energy Medicine Daily Energy Routine *(https://edenenergymedicine.com/#)*

The *Cross Crawl exercise* included in Eden's daily energy routine balances and harmonizes energy, improves coordination, and clears thinking and is done as follows:

1. *While standing, sitting, or lying down, lift your right arm and left leg simultaneously.*

2. *As you let them down, raise your left arm and right leg.*

3. *Repeat, this time exaggerating the lift of your leg and the swing of your arm across the midline to the opposite side of your body.*

4. *If you can, twist so that your elbow touches your opposite knee.*

5. *Continue for at least a minute, breathing deeply in through your nose and out through your mouth.*

Dr. Titus Chiu, Functional Neurologist and author of BrainSAVE! (http://drtituschiu.com/)

To improve balance and coordination:

1. *Balance on your left foot as long as you can and then on your right foot as long as you can. The one on which you can stand the shortest amount of time is your least coordinated side.*

2. *Do the balance exercise on the side that is the least coordinated by standing and balancing on this leg with the other leg raised off the floor.*

3. *This exercise strengthens your base of support and fine-tunes the ability of the nerve fibers responsible for balance to determine your body's positioning in space.*

Exercises to Improve Posture

12 Exercises to Improve Posture: https://www.healthline.com/health/posture-exercises#child's-pose-

Having good posture is about more than looking good. It helps you to develop strength, flexibility, and balance in your body. Proper posture also reduces stress on your muscles and ligaments, which can reduce your risk of injury.

Posture Exercise #1 – Isometric Rows

1. Sit in a chair with a soft back.

2. Bend your arms so your fingers are facing forward and your palms are facing each other.

3. Exhale as you draw your elbows back into the chair behind you, squeeze your shoulder blades together, and relax your shoulders.

4. Breathe deeply as you hold this position for ten seconds.

5. On an inhale, slowly release to the starting position.

6. Repeat this movement for one minute.

7. Do this exercise several times throughout the day.

Posture Exercise #2 – Child Pose

This resting pose stretches and lengthens your spine, glutes, and hamstrings and helps to release tension in your lower back and neck.

1. Sit on your shinbones with your knees together, your big toes touching, and your heels splayed out to the side.

2. Fold forward at your hips and walk your hands out in front of you.

3. Sink your hips back down toward your feet. If your thighs won't go all the way down, place a pillow or folded blanket under them for support.

4. Gently place your forehead on the floor or turn your head to one side.

5. Keep your arms extended or rest them along your body.

6. Breathe deeply into the back of your rib cage and waist.

7. Relax in this pose for up to five minutes while continuing to breathe deeply.

Other Exercise Suggestions

Warm-up is non-negotiable!

Chris Freytag, Certified Personal Trainer and founder of Get Healthy U TV

Chris Freytag says that warm-up exercises that literally warm your muscles and increase levels of key enzymes to improve fitness performance are important in all stages in life. But warm-up is especially critical the older you get to help prevent joint and muscle injury.

Dancing, the "Star" of Exercise

Have fun dancing while maintaining brain and body fitness! Studies have shown that the elderly experience the most marked improvements in the body and brain from dance therapy. Dancing is considered a psychosocial intervention and combines in one activity a myriad of benefits that include mood-elevation from increased social interaction and improvements in brain function and quality of life.

Strength Training

Cindy Anderson, Certified Personal Trainer and Fitness Director, Professional Fitness Center in Copiague, New York

Anderson says that "one of the best forms of cardiovascular exercise for older adults is walking." Recommended are the following:

1. *Start with 5 to 10 minutes of light walking three to four times per week*

2. *Gradually work up to 20 to 30 minutes of brisk walking five times per week.*

Swimming

Victoria Shin, MD, Cardiologist, Torrance Memorial Medical Center, California

Swimming is called the world's perfect exercise. "Getting in the pool is a great way to increase your cardiovascular fitness while also strengthening your muscles," says Dr. Victoria Shin, and it puts minimal stress on your bones and joints. A 2012 study published in the Journal of Aging Research suggests that swimming can help older adults keep their minds as sharp as their bodies.

Pilates

Pilates is known for being a low-impact strength program that focuses on core strength and stability, which is great for older adults. An analysis published in the European Review of Aging and Physical Activity in 2014 concluded that Pilates improves balance in older adults.

Yoga

David Kruse, MD, Sports Medicine Specialist, Hoag Orthopedic Institute, Orange, California

Yoga helps build muscle strength, aerobic fitness, balance, core stability, mobility and flexibility—"all of which are important for older adults," says Dr. David Kruse. Yoga is low-impact and gentle on the body's joints but also is weight-bearing, vital to strengthening not just your muscles, but also your bones.

- SilverSneakers — **https://www.silversneakers.com/class/yoga**

Adding even one or two yoga poses to your daily routine can help your mobility and reduce the risk of falls and injuries.

Mountain Pose – This is an active pose that improves posture, balance, and calm focus and exercises every muscle in the body. It is also helpful for reducing back pain and relieving sciatica.

1. *Stand with your feet hip-width apart.*
2. *Roll your shoulders up, back, and down.*
3. *Stand tall, feeling your feet rooted into the ground.*
4. *Breathe deeply for three to five breaths.*

- *Easier – do the pose sitting tall in a chair.*
- *Harder – lift your arms straight up to the sky or lift your heels to challenge your balance.*

Tree Pose – Excellent pose to work on balance, reducing the risk of falls.

1. *Stand in mountain pose with your feet, knees and hips facing forward.*
2. *Shift your weight to your right foot. Turn you left toes slightly out.*
3. *Lift your heel and draw it toward your right foot like a kickstand.*
4. *Draw your belly in for support and stand tall.*
5. *Breathe for three to five breaths.*
6. *Return to mountain pose and repeat on the other side.*
   - *Easier – keep your feet facing the same direction or only lift your heel slightly.*
   - *Harder – place the sole of your lifted foot inside the calf of your standing leg.*

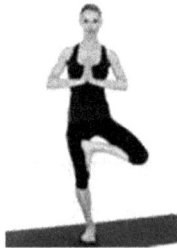

- Video exercises can be found on Collage: https://www.collagevideo.com/.
- A free 28 day beginners' yoga program can be found at https://www.doyouyoga.com/the-10-most-important-yoga-poses-for-beginners-25270/

- Great posture and other exercises as well as access to other tips (makeup, etc.) for seniors can be found on YouTube. https://www.youtube.com/watch?v=WJspJaFL_l8&has_verified=1 and https://eldergym.com/exercises/.

My Exercise Program

Gym

I go to the gym three times a week, working out most days for 45–50 minutes. Because of knee and leg problems, I ride the stationary bike for only 10–15 minutes. However, I incorporate interval training, which is an added burst of harder or faster exercise alternating with easier or slower exercise. The interval workout reaps the same rewards that would be accomplished with a longer workout. Following is my interval program for riding the stationary bike:

1. *I measure my heart rate as I begin.*

2. *I peddle fast with my arms moving from side to side over my head for 90 seconds.*

3. *Then I peddle slowly with my arms down and motionless for 60 seconds and repeat this sequence for 10 minutes, measuring my heart rate after each high-intensity cycle.*

   Generally, my heart rate will have increased between 30 and 40 beats. This interval training involving high-intensity exercise is highly effective in conditioning the cardiovascular system while increasing muscle strength. Active rest between high-intensity exercises allows the heart rate to drop, giving the body the opportunity to recover before the next high-intensity interval. Raising my arms increases my heart rate significantly, slims my waist, and helps facilitate an interval aerobic exercise that results in the same fitness as a longer session. (This multi-tasking also makes my Type-A personality happy!!!)

4. *After riding the bike, I use the machines that focus on every area of my body: abdomen, lower and upper back, shoulders, arms, and legs.*

5. *Then, I go through the 10 stretches on the Precor Stretch Trainer (shown below), which stretches every part of the body to increase flexibility, mobility, and reduce muscle tension.*

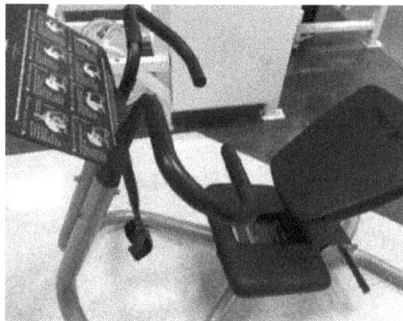

6. *I jump on a miniature trampoline for a count of 100 to rev up the circulation of my lymphatic and blood systems.*

7. *I follow with freestanding exercises to stretch my Achilles tendon, quadriceps, and lower back.*

8. *Lastly, I walk around the track a couple of times.*

9. *I then take my blood pressure, which is generally a healthy twenty points lower than when I started.*

My stamina and energy and brain repair have increased as a result of my dedication to exercise—and I'm looking good!

Home Workout

The Eden Energy Medicine Daily Energy Routine

On days when I do not go to the gym, I take 5–7 minutes to do Donna Eden's daily energy routine, which helps to establish positive "energy habits" in the body that strengthen the immune system and help reduce stress. Go to Eden's website for a free video that shows how to perform the **Daily Energy Routine** (https://edenenergymedicine.com/donnas-daily-energy-routine/) or order **The Little Book of Energy Medicine** or **The Daily Routine Handout** (https://edenenergymedicine.com/product-category/all-products/page/3/).

Dr. Titus Chiu's BrainSAVE!

In his book ***BrainSAVE!***, Dr. Chiu gives quizzes to determine which part of the brain needs repair and then recommends exercises that help heal the affected section of the brain. After a couple of weeks of doing these exercises, I noticed improvement in my cognitive function, my coordination, and my positive outlook and motivation. Great book!!!

I highly recommend that everyone check out the above activities and, with your doctor's approval, incorporate them in your daily exercise routine.

Confidence Feeling Vibration Platform

I have a platform that shakes my body as I stand on it for ten minutes. It purportedly does the following:

- Increases muscle strength
- Improves circulation
- Improves general fitness

- Increases bone density
- Combats cellulite

If you suffer from joint problems, have a heart condition, or use a pacemaker, the company that makes the platform recommends seeking medical advice before using a vibration trainer. This machine is highly rated by customers, but frankly, I have not used it consistently enough to be a good source for recommending it or affirming its benefits.

Strength Exercises

During an appointment with **Dr. Craig Castanet** for decompression therapy, he showed me strength exercises using weights. He recommends weight lifting each day as the best exercise to keep the body and mind healthy. I incorporate these in my exercise program at the gym. (http://backstrong.net/services/ergonomics-videos/)

The American College of Sports Medicine now recommends weight training for all people over 50, and even for people well into their 90s. A group of nursing home residents ranging from ages 87 to 96 improved their muscle strength by almost 180 percent after just eight weeks of weight lifting, also known as strength training. Adding that much strength is almost like rolling back the clock. Even frail elderly people find their balance improves, their walking pace quickens, and stairs become less of a challenge.

> **For information and exercises specifically for seniors:**
> https://www.silversneakers.com/blog/strength-training-for-seniors/

To maintain youthful energy, improve your health, increase your longevity, and look younger than your age, exercise is essential. Choose the exercises that cover all bases: aerobic fitness, physical strength, and brain and body health . . . and make a commitment to do them daily—WITHOUT FAIL! In the next section, learn brain regeneration techniques, followed by supplementation.

Brain Regeneration Techniques

Mental Practices

Exercising your mind as suggested herein is a great way to keep it sharp. You can stimulate the mind by learning new things, reading, listening to music, interacting with others, and exploring.

> One activity that has been shown to be clearly destructive to the brain is watching too much TV; therefore, for continued brain health, it is important to limit the time you spend idly in front of the screen.

A 2011 study published in the ***Journal of Neuropsychiatry*** found that activities such as playing games and crafting, such as quilting and knitting, reduced rates of cognitive impairment by up to 50 percent. Engaging in art also ranks high on the list of brain-healthy hobbies. Studies prove that, once again, it's not enough to be a passive observer.

Practices to Enhance Your Mind

1. **Take a nature walk** - University of Michigan researchers found that memory and attention improved 20 percent when people walked in a

park versus an urban environment. Natural settings have a restful effect, allowing the brain to better process information.

2. **Tai Chi** - Studies have long shown that tai chi improves balance. Research now demonstrates it may also protect the area of the brain responsible for the sense of touch, which fades rapidly after age 40.

3. **Sprint** – A study found that exercisers who did a 3-minute sprint memorized new words 20 percent faster because sprinting triggered growth in the hippocampus, the area responsible for memory and verbal learning. https://www.ncbi.nlm.nih.gov/pmc/articles/PMC4929070/

4. **Exercise** - In a Canadian study, older adults who lifted weights along with walking and balance exercises improved their decision-making abilities by nearly 13 percent in 6 months.

   a. **Balancing Arm Raise** - stand holding dumbbells at sides, palms back. Lift right knee to hip height as you raise left arm up in front, elbow straight, until its overhead. Lower and switch sides.

   b. **Ballerina Curl** - stand with feet wide, toes out, holding dumbbells at sides, palms forward. Bend knees, lowering hips. As you stand, curl dumbbells toward shoulders and lift heels. Lower dumbbells, then heels, and repeat.

   c. **Coordination Crunch** - Lie on back with a dumbbell in each hand near chest, elbows bent out to sides, legs extended over hips, and abs tight. Simultaneously open legs into a 'V' as you lift your head and shoulders off floor and press weights straight up over chest. Lower to start, bringing legs together, and repeat.

Dr. Brant Cortright (The Neurogenesis Diet and Lifestyle) states that "no size fits all" as far as mental stimulation is concerned. He suggests experimenting with different activities to find what works for you and is not too easy or too hard. Using the mind throughout our lives is like an insurance policy against Alzheimer's and dementia. Included in his suggestions for mental practices that impact the mind are the following:

More Practices to Enhance the Mind

1. Reading – read with variety: fiction (novels and short stories), nonfiction (biography, self-help, inspirational, history), poetry, newspaper and magazine articles, and social media posts.

2. Writing – journal, e-mails, texts, stories, poems, articles, and marketing ads.

3. Attention and concentration – focus on one task at a time and meditate.

4. Executive function tasks – organizing, planning, executing, following through, and completing complex tasks.

5. Discussion groups – expressing thoughts and also hearing and taking in others views.

6. Musical training – learning to play an instrument.

7. Education – new learning, formally or informally.

Supplementation

Determine if your supplements are needed! Before discussing supplements or foods as remedies for aging conditions, let me share with you a procedure that has been invaluable to me in determining the supplements/foods that I need each day.

Morning and evening, I stand with my feet close together and hold the supplement bottle or food (on spoon or fork) against my midsection. If my body sways forward, the product will be beneficial, and if my body sways backward, the product is not currently needed. If products test positive, I determine dosage by holding one tablet, capsule, or dropper against my midsection and increase the number until I no longer get a positive response (forward swaying). The result can change from morning to night and from day to day and is very valuable in regulating what I take. This Middle Eastern practice has been accurate and of great value for me in determining the supplements and quantity to take each day.

Supplements can be of great benefit to your brain's health but I want to emphasize that the most important thing you can do for your brain is to eat a nutritious, natural diet.

> Supplements are not magic bullets that will repair and create brain cells if you are eating a crappy diet that includes excessive sugar, high-fructose corn syrup, too many calories, trans fats, and processed and pesticide-laden foods.

Cleaning up your diet is imperative before considering taking supplements.

Brain Cell Health

The first thing to realize is that the brain is always under construction, even in a person's later years. Therefore, it is important to feed the brain with the proper building materials, including nourishing foods and supplements, and to discover if you are deficient in important nutrients.

Highly publicized recently has been that the majority of Americans have deficiencies of vitamin D and magnesium, nutrients that effect your brain. Ask your doctor to test your levels of these substances to ensure that their levels are adequate in your body.

Omega-3 (DHA) is also critical to your brain health and your happiness. It promotes growth and activates and nourishes the part of your brain that makes you happy and peaceful. A Tufts University study found that high levels of DHA decrease memory and brain problems by 47 percent. DHA prevents your brain from shrinking as you get older! Foods containing high levels of omega-3s are fish (such as salmon, tuna, and halibut) and other seafood (including algae and krill), as well as cod liver oil, flax, chia, and walnuts.

Stress is very toxic to the brain because of the high levels of cortisol it produces. The cortisol negatively impacts the brain's memory center, the hippocampus, and the gut. Surprisingly, a way to lower the level of cortisol in your body is to consciously smile! Also, let go of judgment! Negative judgments of people you encounter increases cortisol, but the act of smiling provides benefits to your brain and body. Simple, but possibly life changing!

Alzheimer's disease and/or Dementia Remedy

*Dr. Mary Newport, a board-certified doctor in pediatrics and neonatology, founding director of the newborn intensive care unit at Spring Hill Regional Hospital in Florida, and clinical faculty assistant professor at the University of South Florida, reported in an interview for the **Awakening From Alzheimer's** series that she was devastated when her husband, Steve, developed symptoms of Alzheimer's disease. Steve, an accountant, was only 52 years old when he was diagnosed with early-onset Alzheimer's! He quickly deteriorated to a point where he couldn't function and the drugs the neurologist put him on didn't change his condition. Steve was not accepted in clinical trials of experimental drugs because his condition was so severe.*

Dr. Newport was not willing to let her husband slip away, and so she frequently researched late into the night searching for something that might help him. She was convinced that there was an answer and relentlessly searched for something that worked. Finally, she discovered a "medical food" that gave her hope: half the patients on the medical food in the study showed memory improvement.

The "medical food" MCT Oil, a medium-chain triglyceride, that is the main component in coconut oil.

Dr. Newport immediately drove to the health food store and bought a jar of non-hydrogenated extra-virgin coconut oil. She then added two teaspoons of coconut oil to Steve's oatmeal, and the results were stunning. At his doctor's appointment that same day, Steve scored 28 percent higher than he had on the previous day! On day 37 of taking coconut oil, the light bulb in Steve's brain switched on. A miracle had happened—Steve was back!

The benefit of coconut oil and MCT is from forming ketones, a high-energy brain fuel. Brain neurons start to die without a constant supply of glucose, which is supplied in their absence by ketones. You might remember that the famous low-carb, high-protein Atkins diet produced ketones and was promoted for weight loss because the body burns fat instead of carbohydrates. Since then, scientists have been studying the effects of ketones on the brain.

Dr. Newport's website has links to twenty scientific papers documenting the positive effect of ketones on mental function.
https://coconutketones.com/

Dr. Newport's Recommendations:

- *Mix 16 ounces of MCT oil with 12 ounces of coconut oil and store at room temperature so it will stay liquid. The level of ketones in coconut oil increases slowly and peaks from three to seven hours after consumption, and MCT oil peaks around 90 minutes, so you get the benefit of both by adding them together. Take a half teaspoon to one teaspoon, especially with MCT oil. Increase over two or three days and work up to 4–6 tablespoons a day (or even more, divided over two to four meals.) Dr. Newport got Steve up to ten or eleven tablespoons a day using a combination of straight coconut oil or MCT and coconut oil together—but it took months to get to that level.*

- *For those in medical facilities, the drug "Axona," a medical grade MCT, is available by prescription. Dr. Newport says the FDA has approved one dose a day but thinks people would need three or four doses a day to sustain ketones around the clock.*

- *To incorporate more MCT or coconut oil in your diet, mix either or both in many foods. Be aware that if you overwhelm your digestive system with too much oil too fast, you might experience indigestion, cramps, or diarrhea. [Note: If I take over one tablespoon of MCT each day, I get digestive distress, including stomach pains and diarrhea.]*

My Suggestions:

- *Mix coconut oil or MCT with freshly ground almond butter.*

- *Soften butter (preferably organic) or ghee at room temperature and add coconut oil or MCT oil in an equal amount. Add to soups, veggies, etc.*

- *Cook with coconut oil but at not more than 350 degrees because high heat will alter the fat, destroying the ketones.*

- *Add one teaspoon to one tablespoon of MCT in coffee — it is tasteless. I add several shakes of ground cinnamon to the mixture and get the benefit of creating a pleasant taste while positively influencing my blood sugar.*

- *Make salad dressings from coconut or MCT oil or add either to existing salad dressings.*

- *Add coconut or MCT oil to smoothies.*

There are many natural substances that encourage or promote brain health but I will only include those listed in **Dr. Titus Chiu's book *BrainSAVE!*, Dr. Brant Cortright's book, *The Neurogenesis Diet & Lifestyle***, and **Dr. Dan Engle's *The Concussion Repair Manual*** because these books provide information that I trust and with which I am impressed. My suggestion for you is to conduct research with your own sources that you trust.

Brain Supplements

Recommended by Dr. Titus Chiu in BrainSAVE!:

- DHA – fatty acid found in brain

- Magnesium L-threonate – a type of magnesium that crosses the blood brain barrier to stabilize unstable brain cells

- Liposomal glutathione – the brain's master antioxidant

- Ginkgo Biloba – improves circulation to brain cells and protects the brain from stress-induced cell death

- Curcumin – natural anti-inflammatory

Partial List of Supplements recommended by Dr. Brant Cortright in The Neurogenesis Diet & Lifestyle (in addition to what's listed in the Diet section):

- Omega-3s (DHA) – most important nutrient for brain health and to promote neurogenesis

- Ginseng extract – increases brain cell creation, protects the brain from injury and stroke, enhances memory, and is an antidepressant

- Quercetin – has anti-inflammatory and antioxidant effects

- DHEA and pregnenolone – "youth hormones"

- Rhodiola – stimulates neurogenesis

- Melatonin – increases neurogenesis and regulates it and increases immunity

- Lithium – provides neuroprotective benefit from brain shrinkage

Partial List of Supplements from Dr. Dan Engle's The Concussion Repair Manual:

Dr. Engle recommends biologic nootropics, a "class of 'smart' drugs and supplements used to enhance brain function."

- Phosphatidylserine (PS) and Phosphatidylcholine (PC) – play an essential role in neuron survival and recovery from injury

- Glutathione (GSH) – eases oxidative stress, contributor to cell signaling and the immune system

- Vitamin C – an important antioxidant in the brain

- B12 (Methylcobalamin) – strong neuroregenerative property

- Acetyl-L-Carnitine (ALC) – improves spatial recognition, judgment, and mood stability and better memory and social skills.

> Have fun as you stimulate your mind by choosing to do some of the practices herein that you enjoy.

Continue on to the next section to understand how spiritual practices influence your mind.

The Spiritual Connection

Perhaps you are questioning what a "spiritual connection" has to do with anti-aging. *Everything!!* In the past, very little scientific research was done on spirituality because of the difficulty assessing it in a concrete way; however, recently, neuroscientists have been able to investigate the effects of spiritual practices on the brain and have found evidence that spiritual practices stimulate neurogenesis (production of new brain cells). For instance, it has been proven that meditation or prayer (that is, stillness or quiet sitting) are dynamic and appear to stimulate the production of brain cells. In this chapter, you will learn ways to enhance your spiritual connection.

On the contrary, researchers Kenneth Pargament and Harold Koenig found that those who experience religious or spiritual discontent have shortened life spans. These included people who believed God was punishing them, had guilt and fear, or had negative attitudes toward God, clergy or other church members.

Before we go further, let me say that the research I've studied does not promote or recommend a particular religion or spiritual practice; instead, it recognizes that being involved in any positive spiritual path or practice enhances a person's brain and increases longevity.

Andrew Newberg, MD and Mark Robert Waldman relate in their book *How God Changes Your Brain: Breakthrough Findings from a Leading Neuroscientist* that from the moment we encounter God or the idea of God, our brain begins to change. They conclude that "the more we engage in spiritual practices, the more control we gain over our body, mind, and fate." Listed below are some of these authors' beneficial activities for maintaining a healthy brain:

1. Faith: Faith is equivalent with hope, optimism, and the belief that a positive future awaits us.

2. Dialogue with others: The more social ties we have, the less cognitive abilities will decline.

3. Meditate: Visualization, guided imagery, and self-hypnosis are specific variations of meditation and are equally effective in maintaining a healthy brain.

4. Yawn: It not only relaxes you but also quickly brings you into a "heightened" state of cognitive awareness.

5. Consciously relax: This refers to deliberately scanning each part of your body to reduce muscle tension and physical fatigue. This exercise increases calmness of the mind and allows the brain to rejuvenate.

6. Stay intellectually active: Intellectual and cognitive stimulation strengthens the neural connections and improves your ability to communicate, solve problems, and make rational decisions concerning your behavior.

7. Smile: The act of smiling repetitively helps interrupt mood disorders and strengthen the brain's neural ability to maintain a positive outlook on life.

How many of the above practices can you truly say you do daily? Certainly you yawn!

Meditate

Meditation is one of the most beneficial spiritual practices for the brain and body and is beneficial in the following ways:

1. Increases the growth of new brain cells

2. Increases your IQ

3. Improves your mental focus, memory, and decision making

4. Reduces stress, anxiety, depression, and irritability

> If you want to remain young in body, mind, and spirit, add a meditation practice to your daily routine.

Three beneficial meditations that I have done or am doing are:

1. *The Soul of Healing Meditations: A Simple Approach to Growing Younger* by Deepak Chopra: www.Amazon.com/theSoulofHealingMeditations. Dr. Chopra takes one through ways to heal the body with the mind. (I love his soothing voice.)

2. *Guided Healing Meditation with Patrick from Samarpan Foundation, Goa, India,* a Biogetica Meditation (free): http://www.biogetica.com/guided-meditations.php. I found the first meditation listed has profoundly influenced my sense of well-being and motivation. The presenter says that this meditation is different in that it focuses outward rather than inward. I only listen to 20 minutes or so of this 51-minute meditation, which takes me through surrounding my family and friends with love and other positive feelings.

3. *Love, Gratitude and Forgiveness, Brain Entrainment and Rich Words to Enhance Your Life Experience* by Keith Scott-Mumby, MD, PhD - www.advancedmindstrategies.com/. Dr. Scott-Mumby takes you through positive events that initiate happiness and eliminate negativity.

At the end of this chapter, Samuel Fernandez Carriba, PhD, a Senior Psychologist in Atlanta, GA, has written important information about meditation and the influence it has had on his life. Please refer to this for more in-depth information.

My Experience of Faith

Following is my story of how a spiritual practice changed, perhaps even saved, my life:

Sukyo Mahikari (True Light) is a practice that I have been a part of for over 32 years. It is not a religion but can be incorporated into all religions to purify the soul and bring people closer to God. As a result, it heals the mind and body. (It is recognized by the United Nations as an international interfaith organization that aims to promote peace and harmony in society through spiritual purification and practice of universal principles such as gratitude, acceptance of the will of God, and humility.)

A friend of mine who was a Christian minister became a member of Sukyo Mahikari and said his parishioners asked him why he would belong to this group. His reply was, "Because it enhances my religion."

Many years ago, someone at a Unity Church Mastermind Group saw my despair and approached me after the meeting to tell me about "something that might help" me. It was Sukyo Mahikari. At that time, I was experiencing severe depression, taking multiple drugs for hormonal problems, had a close family member in jail, had just gotten divorced, couldn't get a job, had filed for bankruptcy, and was dismissed by my therapist who said she "couldn't help me."

Having been brought up in the Presbyterian Church and even having taught adult Sunday school, I was skeptical upon going to the Sukyo Mahikari Center; it seemed strange and was not like anything I had previously encountered. In fact, I told a friend afterwards that it was the weirdest thing I'd ever experienced and I wasn't going back. However, my friend who did not know this practice or the organization talked me into going back; he knew my desperation. God's arrangement? Absolutely! Consequently, I went back every day for several months because it was relaxing.

I became a member after I was assured "you don't have to believe" because I still wasn't sure it was compatible with my beliefs. However, after a year I reflected on my membership and couldn't deny the positive things that had resulted: my depression had disappeared, and I was able to get off all the hormones I was taking (even though my doctor had said I would have to take the thyroid hormone for the rest of my life), my family member had all criminal charges dropped, I got a job the day after I became a member, and my therapist apologized and said she had meant that only God could help me.

Life got better over the years in a steady step-by-step manner. I found a purpose in life and a spiritual family who substituted for my children and their families who live in a faraway state. Now, I'm happy, and my purpose is to encourage and support all people who enter my life and need help, just as I was helped. My key to happiness is focusing on others rather than focusing on myself and my perceived problems. Thank God for Sukyo Mahikari. http://www.sukyomahikari.org/

The message to take away from this chapter is that involvement in a spiritual activity helps keep the brain healthy. Whatever resonates with your beliefs and makes your life better is the spiritual connection that is right for you. Enhance your life in this way!

Read on for Samuel's story.

Practicing "Health and Happiness Through Meditation"

My good friend **Samuel Fernandez Carriba, PhD,** a clinical psychologist at a major university in Atlanta, GA, does assessments and diagnosis with special needs children as well as meditation training with their families and providers. Equally important, he is one of the most loving and compassionate people I've ever known. For that reason, and because he inspires me, I asked him to write about what he thinks is important for leading a long, healthy, fulfilling life. He graciously agreed.

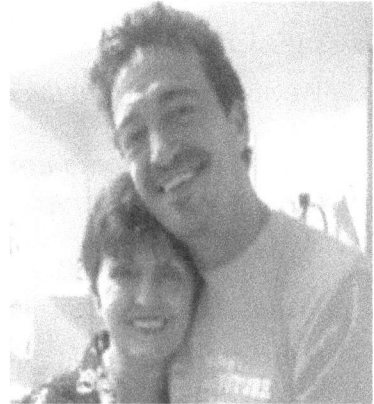

Following is Samuel's story as he tells it:

Let me tell you a little bit about myself. I'm a sensitive person that easily gets overwhelmed. I'm a great planner that quickly falls into anxiety. These are my virtues and my flaws, depending on the situation and of whom you ask. As I studied psychology, I learned about those principles that make a person healthy and happy. I felt powerful with all that knowledge but also increasingly disappointed at myself for seeming incapable so often of practicing what was otherwise so clear. I felt a little bit like an addict, doing often the opposite of what I was supposed to do and not being able to help it. Then, I felt the weight of shame at this realization. Every new life crisis, whether graduating, changing jobs, or a romantic break-up, led me to clinical depression. Then, at age 34, I was diagnosed with brain cancer.

The point here is that, although we can and we should learn general principles about well-being and health, the devil, and God if I may, are in the detail. There are always exceptions to the rule and sometimes these exceptions may be more important than the rule itself (i.e., the point where being a great planner leads to distress). The only way to know those details in each concrete situation is through experience, through practice: knowing most of the rules is helpful but not sufficient to be healthy and happy. We must practice. We must make mistakes. We must learn from the mistakes. And then continue to practice.

When I fell into the umpteenth episode of depression after being declared in complete remission from my cancer, desperate as I was, I allowed a friend to convince me to try "meditation" as part of a research study at Emory University. Meditation, my friend told me, could be defined simply as "mind training" and it did not have to be spiritual or religious, which was important for me at the time. It is actually compatible with any religious or spiritual practice or with none. It was the year 2007, which was not the first time the American public had paid attention to meditation but the beginning of a series of scientific studies that led to journalist Dan B. Harris reporting on ABC news in 2015: "I think we are looking at meditation as the next health revolution."

Now, meditation is becoming just that, a health revolution, exceeding all expectations about benefits in physical and mental health across the board. As described in helpguide.org, meditation can: help relieve stress, treat heart disease, lower blood pressure, reduce chronic pain, improve sleep, and alleviate gastrointestinal difficulties. In recent years, psychotherapists have also turned to mindfulness meditation as an important element in the treatment of a number of problems, including: depression, substance abuse, eating disorders, couples' conflicts, anxiety disorders, and obsessive-compulsive disorder. Meditation is then mental training, but what do we exactly train when we meditate?

Although there are different styles of meditation practice, mindful awareness is an essential component in all. According to Jon Kabat-Zin, generally considered the person behind the popularity of mindfulness in its modern context, it is precisely about "how" we pay attention: purposefully, in the present moment, and nonjudgmentally. There is a second group of analytical practices, built upon mindfulness but going beyond the non-conceptual exercise, in which this purposeful attention is used for introspection or reflection on the contents of the mind. One example of an analytical meditation practice is "compassion" meditation, in which a series of exercises specifically promote compassion, or the desire and engaged action to alleviate suffering, toward self and others.

Shauna Shapiro and collaborators published an article in 2006 entitled "Mechanisms of Mindfulness" in which they described these three axioms of mindfulness: attention, intention, and attitude. In both types of analytical and non-conceptual practices, "what" is trained is attention, a skill that is necessary for absolutely everything that we do. Attention is synonymous with awareness for psychologists. This is an ability described by the father of American psychology, William James, as very difficult to train: "It is easier to define this ideal than to give practical directions for bringing it about." Axiom 2, the intention, is our purpose, "why" we practice, and ultimately, why we live. Although a very personal question, human beings are more similar than different about this. Whether your answer is happiness, peace, flourishing, if we were to ask the 7 billion of people in the planet, "do you want to feel better or worse," guess what the unanimous answer will be.

Together with the what (the attention) and the why (the intention), there is a third element in this practice, which I will call the "how," or the attitude. Jon Kabat-Zin defines this attitude as non-judgmental. It is the kind but honest non-judgmental attitude that we apply to how we do things. It is an attitude of equanimity, of balance, of applying not too much exertion but not too little effort, just enough to get us what we want at a reasonable cost. In a most basic example in real life, there is an ideal point between overworking, being burnout, and staying all day in bed doing nothing. Where is our health and our happiness? It is in the balance between what we invest and what we get.

The "how" is the harder element in the practice to define and describe, but present in all the compassion meditation protocol that I started to practice in 2007. I have now been using it for five years with families of individuals with autism and providers (and many others) to help them reduce their stress and increase their resiliency. Compassion meditation training takes the participant through a series of sequential exercises which start with simple breathing, then attention exercises, and continues with very personal but also universal questions about what it is that we want in life and how to get closer to it. In this search for health and well-being, it is key to bring awareness to how we relate to ourselves and to others, and that is why the word compassion is part of it. A simple exercise that I sometimes share with people who take the course follows.

> *Imagine that you are about to leave a room and somebody you don't know slams the door in your face.*
>
> *(Pause)*
>
> *What are your thoughts? What are your feelings? What is your opinion of this person?*
>
> *(Pause)*
>
> *Now, consider each one of these possible scenarios, given that you know very little to nothing about this person and their circumstances. After reading each one, pause for a moment and assess your overall physiological state. Feel free to elaborate on imaginary details in each one of them that help you figure out how you are feeling.*
>
> - *They could be just plain rude.*
>
>   *(Pause)*
>
> - *They could be absent-minded.*
>
>   *(Pause)*
>
> - *What if they were in a hurry?*

(Pause)

- *What if they were in distress because they just received terrible news?*

(Pause)

Given equally likely possibilities, which option makes your body feel lighter? If you could choose how to feel, how would you choose to feel?

Health and happiness are then all about practice. We need the contents (we need this book!), we need the purpose, and we need to practice.

Compassion meditation is the best framework that I have ever encountered with suggestions on how to apply these contents to our everyday life. Nothing like this mental exercise offers me a strategy to learn how to learn, to recognize which behavior may be the healthiest for me at a certain point and to learn from my mistakes, beyond categories like flaws or virtues.

When I landed into brain cancer the second time in 2016 after practicing this method for nine years, I was really able, with the help of others, to turn around this experience. I say this knowing how strange it sounds, but cancer the second time was a real party. It came and it went. I had a great time with it.

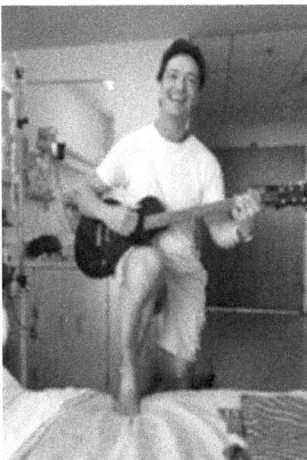

Note from Margianna: I visited Samuel in the hospital many times during the year he was receiving chemo for active brain cancer and couldn't believe what I saw: a young man hooked up to chemo IVs, playing his guitar, singing and dancing! A happy person that appeared not to have a care in the world! Amazingly, he shared his happiness with the other cancer patients on the floor by going from room to room, singing and playing!

Samuel continues: *Even more important for me than being a cancer survivor is being a depression survivor. My depression never came back since 2007. For details about my own personal experience, with details about how to register for the training, you can see a short video in YouTube entitled "The Compassion to Conquer." (https://www.youtube.com/watch?v=mbXxo_oZqsY)*

Samuel is a wonderful role model of one offering a positive influence in this world! Please check out the link and, if you are in the Atlanta area, participate in one of Samuel's compassion trainings. Thank you, Samuel, for being in my life! God is good!

Continue reading to learn next about the role sleep plays in brain health and ways to improve your sleeping habits.

Sleep

Our current lifestyle and the fact that we are a society of overachievers are greatly affecting our ability to get adequate sleep. Unfortunately, skimping on sleep can affect your health in more ways than you might imagine. Are you getting enough sleep so that you wake up invigorated and ready to meet the challenges of the day and, even more importantly, to keep your brain healthy? If not, incorporate the tips in this chapter to get more restful sleep.

Dr. Daniel Amen wrote:

"Getting less than six hours of sleep each night has been associated with lower overall brain activity. When you miss out on sleep, your brain pays the price. Chronic lack of sleep leads to a loss of brain cells and also increases the brain plaque believed to contribute to age-related memory loss and Alzheimer's disease."

Sleep deprivation is hazardous to your health!

David Wolfe and New Horizon Health reports:

A lack of sleep can break down the immune system and harm the adrenal system. Wolfe interestingly says a proper night's sleep is very important for our left brain; but not necessarily for our right brain. Consequently, if you're in a left-brain/analytical type job, you need to get more sleep. [Note: I've never heard this before!]

John Peever, director of the Systems Neurobiology Laboratory at the University of Toronto, and Brian J. Murray, director of the sleep laboratory at the Sunnybrook Health Sciences Center state:

Sleep serves to reenergize the body's cells, clear waste from the brain, and support learning and memory. It even plays vital roles in regulating mood, appetite and libido. Most of the sleeping we do is characterized by large, slow brain waves, relaxed muscles, and slow, deep breathing, which may help the brain and body to recuperate after a long day.

National Institute for Neurological Disorders and Strokes (https://www.ninds. nih.gov/Disorders/Patient-Caregiver-Education/Understanding-Sleep#8)

There is no magic "number of sleep hours" that work for everybody of the same age. Most adults need 7–9 hours of sleep a night, but after age 60, nighttime sleep tends to be shorter, lighter, and interrupted by multiple awakenings.

Elderly people are also more likely to take medications that interfere with sleep.

In general, people are getting less sleep than they need due to longer work hours and the availability of 'round-the-clock entertainment and other activities. Many people feel they can "catch up" on missed sleep during the weekend, but depending on how sleep-deprived they are, sleeping longer on the weekends may not be adequate.

Quality sleep is as essential to survival as food and water. Without sleep you can't form or maintain the pathways in your brain that let you learn and create new memories, and it's harder to concentrate and respond quickly.

Tips to Improve Sleep

- Set a schedule – go to bed and wake up at the same time each day.

- Exercise 20 to 30 minutes a day but no later than a few hours before going to bed.

- Avoid caffeine and nicotine late in the day as well as avoiding alcoholic drinks before bed.

- Relax before bed – try a warm bath, reading, or another relaxing routine.

- Create a room for sleep - avoid bright lights and loud sounds, keep the room at a comfortable temperature, and don't watch TV or have a computer in your bedroom.

- Don't lie in bed awake. If you can't get to sleep, do something else, like reading or listening to music, until you feel tired.

- Meditate before bedtime.

- Investigate supplements that will help relax your body and mind (get your doctor's approval before taking sleep supplements):
  o Melatonin

  o Homeopathic combinations, such as Boiron's Quietude

  o Magnesium

- o GABA

- o Theanine

- o Herbs:

  - Valerian Root helps increase the amount of the neurotransmitter GABA in the brain, which brings about relaxation and calm.

  - Passionflower is actually listed as a tranquilizing herb in Germany to calm and induce sleep.

  - Lemon Balm encourages deeper and more restful sleep, as shown in a German sleep study and, among other benefits, is a brain booster that helps memory and mood!

  - Hops studies show that those who drank non-alcoholic beer with hops actually had improved sleep quality and reduced levels of anxiety.

  - Chamomile is most commonly consumed in the form of tea, and its health benefits are multiple: it's an anti-inflammatory that helps with digestive issues, skin irritations, and sore throat and, of course, is an excellent sleep support supplement.

See a doctor if you continue having a problem sleeping or if you feel unusually tired during the day. Most sleep disorders can be treated effectively without harmful drugs.

For a healthy brain and body, do whatever you need to do to avoid sleep deprivation!

Youthful Voice

Are you identified as an "old person" because of your voice? *Read on to discover how to recreate your young voice, regardless of age.*

Claudio Milstein, associate professor of surgery at Cleveland Clinic Lerner College of Medicine says, "There are a lot of things we can do to rejuvenate a voice even though it may be part of the normal aging process." Milstein further explains that typical signs of aging occur around age 65 and as we get older, we get "thin, breathy voices . . . [and] those are the characteristics that make it sound like a person has an old voice." However, not everyone suffers from a wavering voice as she or he ages.

People who are physically and socially active possess stronger voices, and those who sing maintain robust voices throughout their lives. "Voices carry something about the emotional state and health of the body," says Milstein. Previously, healthcare professionals referred those suffering from wavering voices to an ear, nose, and throat (ENT) doctor and recommended they seek help at a voice clinic. Experts recommended speech therapy first, with more serious treatments such as injections or surgery if therapy fails. However, the real answer for maintaining a strong, young-sounding voice is to adopt the healthy lifestyle given in this book.

A youthful voice is another good reason to maintain a healthy diet and exercise your brain and body.

Consciously exercise your voice daily. Some ideas follow.

1. Sing familiar songs loud and clear for at least 10 minutes! (Look in mirror and pretend you are a Broadway star.)

2. Sing scales – high and low notes for 5 minutes.

3. Gargle with warm water for as long as you can, preferably 60 seconds. (Activates the vagus nerve located in the brain stem, resulting in better digestion, calmness and healing. — *BrainSAVE!* by Dr. Titus Chiu)

4. Use your voice as much as possible:

   a. Talk with conviction (forcefully) throughout the day, even if it is to yourself or to the TV!

   b. Call at least one family member or friend each day.

Now that you have a sharp mind, healthy body, are sleeping like a baby, and have a strong, powerful voice, continue in the next section with the following anti-aging information concerning your appearance.

Section Three

~

Look Good
to
Feel Good

Hello, Beautiful!

I have heard women say, "I'm proud of my wrinkles—I've earned them." Excuse me? Not me!!! OK, maybe I'm vain ... however, I choose to think it is because I admire beauty!

Suffice to say, each woman is different and will determine her own priorities. To some, appearance is important and they might say, "I can't go to the mailbox without makeup, coifed hair, and dressed for the day." To others, comfort is the only important consideration and might say, "I'll slip out to mailbox in my robe and slippers." To even others, "No one cares how I look when I get the mail."

What you consider important about your appearance is not all learned choices but also innate preferences. **Neuro-linguistic Programming (NLP — Science of the Mind)** reports that how you take in, process, and put out information is an inborn characteristic. If this is true, then each of us functions from a primary "representational type"—that is, Visual, Auditory, or Kinesthetic. Let me hasten to add that each of us uses all systems but generally tends to favor one over the others and a particular one in specific situations.

So, why do I bring this up now? Our mode of perception or representational type not only influences how we function, including communication and learning, but also what is important to us in our appearance. See if you can identify your primary representational type by the following partial descriptions:

Visual - sight, mental imagery, spatial awareness

- Organized, neat, and well-groomed because it's important to look good.

- Appreciates and is concerned about beauty that is reflected in an attractive outward appearance made up of matching clothes, enhancing cosmetics, and styled hair.

- Fast-paced – speaking, gestures, actions.

- Interested in global goals rather than detailed plans.

- Uses words: look, notice, imagine, picture, and visualize.

- Uses phrases: I see what you mean; We see eye to eye; Show me what you mean; It appears to me.

Auditory/Hearing - sound, speech, dialogue, white noise

- Couldn't care less how they look or if their colors are coordinated or if their patterns match.

- Attracted to music and prefers receiving information or books in audio form. (Have the best quality speakers for their music systems.)

- Volume, tone, and tempo are important.

- Words often used: say, loud, resonate, ring, ask, vocal, speechless, and harmonious.

- Uses phrases: On the same wavelength; Turn a deaf ear; Clear as a bell; Living in harmony.

Kinesthetic/Touch/Feeling - internal feelings in the body

- Dress and groom more for comfort than look.

- Slow to speak and respond.

- Determine how they "feel" inwardly before making a decision or expressing an opinion.

- Words often used: touch, contact, push, warm, cold, sensitive, gentle, heavy, and smooth.

- Phrases used: I will get in touch with you; I can grasp that idea; I feel it in my bones; Heated argument; Scratch the surface.

Neutral

- Words used: decide, think, remember, recognize, understand, process, learn, consider.

Frankly, the representational system you identify with will determine your interest in this section of the book. I confess I am very Visual, so I've devoted a lot of time and effort to find ways to improve my facial and body appearance and to find attractive clothes. I trust this will be helpful to some of you.

Identify your primary representational type:
Visual ____ Auditory ____ Kinesthetic ____ ?

As a Visual, it has always been important to me to maintain a body weight that enhances my appearance. However, I have never believed in dieting. Check out my book ***Unleash the Thin Within: The Spirit, Mind and Body Solution to Permanent Weight Control*** on Amazon or my website, www.unleashthethinwithin.com, to learn how I have controlled my weight (and so can you) without dieting.

Wrinkles, Be Gone!

Face it! The first thing most people notice about you is your face and, from this, make an instant judgment about who you are—that is, are you energetic, happy, interesting, healthy, and/or intelligent or, heaven forbid, *old*. Yes, your crow's feet, sagging jowls, and the deep, dark hollows under your eyes can seriously undermine who you are.

Nothing says "old" like sagging skin!

Cosmetics can hide some of your flaws, but eating a healthy diet (I can't repeat this often enough) is essential to a more youthful look, as well as exercising your face and using transforming and rejuvenating skincare products.

> *"Poor-quality foods, like trans fats, cause inflammation—and aging is basically a chronic inflammatory state," says **Timothy Harlan, MD, assistant professor of medicine at Tulane University School of Medicine**. "Can you look older because you're eating crap? Absolutely."*

(Because of its importance, another section is devoted to what you put in your mouth and yet another to recipes that contribute to health and a youthful look.)

So, what about wrinkles and sagging skin? Facial muscles can lose their normal healthy tone as we grow older because the muscles become too loose or too tight. When the muscles are not toned, they are not healthy and the blood and lymph vessels cannot circulate freely in the face. The result is wrinkles, dry skin, and a lack of skin color. Additionally, the lips grow thinner and the nose grows longer and wider. It is important to realize that your health and longevity as well as your appearance are affected by exercise, including facial exercises. Your face begs for exercise just as your body does—an old, wrinkled look is not inevitable (or desirable)!

Toned muscles in the face result in increased blood circulation and oxygen flow throughout the skin and facial muscles that will:

- Shorten and narrow the enlarged nose
- Plump the lips for a fuller look
- Diminish, if not eliminate, under-eye puffiness
- Tighten the neck skin

Facial exercises can be strengthened with "mindful breathing," that is, focusing on the inhale and exhale as you breathe. In and of itself, mindful breathing enhances youth, beauty, and health, so pay attention to your breathing throughout the day as well as when exercising.

My Ritual

Facial Exercises

I have achieved a facelift simply by working the muscles that support and shape my face. Creating better muscle tone in the face will cause the skin to be tauter and firmer-looking, which can also help to reduce the appearance of fine lines and wrinkles on many areas of the face. Every morning for several minutes, I exercise my face to stimulate blood flow and increase facial collagen and muscle tone.

- *Many years ago, my daughter-in-law's sister, Evie, had Bell's palsy, which left one side of her face paralyzed and drooping. However, several months later when I visited my family in a midwestern state, I saw her and was surprised to see that her face was normal and beautiful as always. I was curious, asked her what happened and she responded by showing me an exercise that was instrumental in her recovery and it was to place both hands beside your mouth, push the muscles upward to beside the nose. Simple but effective!*

I saw significant improvements from the above exercise. It made sense to me that if this exercise could repair the damaged muscles from Bell's palsy, it could also tone all the muscles in a sagging and wrinkled face. I added the following to my morning routine.

- *I look in the mirror and pinpoint wrinkles, lines, or sagging skin. After applying face cream, I push up or push up and out depending on the area on which I want to improve. After exercising the muscles, I pat my face and neck vigorously with my fingers to stimulate circulation.*

- *Something else that I do many times a day that creates improvement in muscle tone (and inner happiness) is I smile!*

Other Facial Exercises

Hollows below the eye that cause a "sunken in" appearance

To eliminate the hollow area beneath the eye, it is necessary to build up a "cushion" or "padding" of muscle beneath the skin which has sunken from muscle atrophy.

Isometric Exercise: *10 minutes per day, minimum (more time will produce faster results):*

1. Sit, relax, and look straight ahead.
2. Without moving your head, look upward as high as possible.
3. Try to "nearly" close your eyes while looking upward.

Your eyes should be almost closed, but not completely. Hold this position for 10 minutes without causing your eyes or face to wrinkle. It may be necessary to do this in front of a mirror the first few times in order to avoid wrinkling the face.

Grow facial muscles

As a woman ages, the muscles in her face sag and droop and, as mentioned, need exercise just like the muscles in the body. The muscles respond to exercise by growing in size, just as the body does. The face then fills out, counteracting sagging skin and thinning fat.

> Consistency is extremely important in performing a facial exercise program if you want positive results.

Results can usually be seen within several weeks to several months.

A Northwestern University study reports that doing facial exercises for five months can make you look three years younger. https://news.northwestern.edu/stories/2018/january/facial-exercises-help-middle-aged-women-appear-more-youthful/

Happy Face Yoga by Gary Sikorski *(https://www.happyfaceyoga.com/)*

The exercises in this program are designed to stimulate the fifty-seven muscles of the face, neck, and scalp. Following are sample exercises included:

The Cheek Lifter: Open your mouth to form an "O" and position your upper lip over teeth. Smile to lift check muscles up, and then put your fingers lightly on the top part of the cheek before releasing the cheek muscles to lower them. Lift the cheeks back up. Repeat by lowering and lifting the cheeks.

Happy Cheeks Sculpting: Smile without showing your teeth. Purse your lips together, and then smile, forcing the cheek muscles up. Place your fingers on the corners of the mouth and slide them up to the top of the cheeks, holding for 20 seconds.

The Yoga Facelift by Marie-Veronique Nadeau

This is an exercise for people who work long hours in front of a computer. It helps reduce puffiness around the eyes and soothes the optic nerve and the eye in general.

Palming

1. Sit comfortably with your back straight and eyes closed.

2. Focus on your breath as it moves in and out of your nostrils. Cool air in, warm air out.

3. Rub palms together very fast until they feel warm and place heels of your hands directly over eyeballs.

4. Contract muscles that surround your eyes against the heel of your hands. Contract and release ten times. Rest and repeat five times.

Sites and books with face exercises

- *Facercise* by Carole Maggio

- Danielle Collins Face Yoga Method, http://www.faceyogaexpert.com/

- Five Anti-aging Facial Exercises, https://www.marieclaire.co.uk/beauty/how-to/anti-ageing-facial-exercises-94678

If you are seriously interested in improving your face through exercise, I suggest that you go to one of the above sites or purchase one of the books listed.

Natural and Organic Beauty Products

Face Creams

Being someone that is "Visual" and, therefore interested in appearance, I have tried many face products. What I have found is that some of the expensive ones are no better than the inexpensive ones. For instance, I paid over a hundred dollars for two products, "Lift & Firm Sculpting Cream" and "Crepe Correcting Body Complex," purportedly formulated by doctors that are renowned for working with movie stars. I saw no results from the products and the company representatives did not answer my e-mails requesting the promised money back if not satisfied. Wasted money!

Before telling you the products that I like, be aware that there are many chemicals in beauty products (some listed below), many of which are being absorbed into your body. Here are ten of the most prevalent:

- Parabens
- Synthetic colors
- Fragrance
- Phthalates
- Triclosan
- Sodium lauryl/laureth sulfate (SLS)
- Formaldehyde
- Toluene
- Propylene glycol
- Sunscreen chemicals

Most of the chemicals listed above are toxic to the immune system as well as being endocrine disruptors, skin irritants, and even human carcinogens. Because of the widespread use of these chemicals, it's difficult to avoid all of them.

> You can limit the amount of toxins to which your body is exposed by eating "clean," avoiding chemical-laden processed foods, using creams and cosmetics free from chemicals when possible, drinking plenty of filtered water, and looking for foods and products that are certified organic.

Healthy Natural Products

To locate healthy makeup and other products, go to the following sites or stores:

- www.thegoodtrade.com/features/18-natural-organic-makeup-brands-your-face-will-love-you-for
- http://www.safecosmetics.org/get-the-facts/big-7/
- www.skyorganics.us/
- https://madesafe.org/
- https://www.skincareox.com/ultimate-list-best-organic-makeup-brands-products/
- Amazon.com
- Brick and mortar stores: Sprouts, Whole Foods, Trader Joe's, health food stores

> **Caveat**: Listed below are the creams, lotions, and serums that have worked best for me—but skin types are different and something that works good for me might not work for you. (My skin is paper thin and would be dry if I didn't pamper it.) I have no affiliation with any of the companies or products and receive no compensation for mentioning them here—they are simply products that have worked for me.

My Face Products

First, let me tell you about the products I started using several months ago and am very pleased with the results, in addition to respecting the company. They are DERMA E® brand products, relatively inexpensive skin products. The company's philosophy: "Since 1984, our passion for health, wellness and environmental sustainability has grown strong. We have high ethical standards and never compromise on skin health and safety." Additionally, "…every DERMA E purchase helps to support global communities and the environment."

DERMA E® products:

- Firming DMAE Cleanser with Alpha Lipoic Acid and C-Ester - This sulfate-free cleanser purifies skin while supporting a visibly firmer, softer, smoother complexion.

- Firming DMAE Serum - This skin-firming product contains DMAE, antioxidants Alpha Lipoic Acid and C-Ester, calming Lemon Grass, Chamomile, natural astringents Horsetail and Horse Chestnut to be gentle on skin while encouraging healthy tone and texture.

- Firming DMAE Moisturizer - A skin-firming formula to help visibly firm, lift and smooth skin as it moisturizes.

I bought my first DERMA E products at Sally's Beauty Supply and later found them on the internet.

"Bell Virtu Organic Nourishing Eye Serum" is a product I just recently ordered and began using. It is promoted to deeply moisture, promote cell regeneration, prevent premature aging, reduce skin discoloration, and assist in increasing collagen and elastin levels. The promotion also says it helps with dry, saggy, tired skin and can be used on the face, neck, chest, forearms, back of hands, and cuticles. It only takes a small drop to cover under the eyes and two small drops to cover the whole face. I haven't used it long enough to know if all the claims are true, but in a short time I have noticed some positive changes. ("Globally sourced, ethical products and award-winning standards") https://www.amazon.com/gp/product/B00KGJVVDK/ref=oh_aui_detailpage_o04_s00?ie=UTF8&psc=1

"theCream" is another company I like to support because it is an ethical company, "Internationally Awarded," and their products are natural and contain colostrum. https://www.thecream.com/

"Asterwood Naturals Matrixyl 3000, Argireline Vitamin C" is described as "anti-aging serum with hyaluronic acid" and is a product that I sometimes use at night with good results. (Amazon.com)

"FineVine" Organic Almond Oil is a great product with many uses — provides a "more youthful, radiant complexion, for dark circles removal, eczema and skin rash relief, muscle fatigue and aches, restores shine to hair and eliminates frizz, hair loss, nail care and more." It is unscented, undiluted, and contains no added ingredients.

Other Products I Sometimes Use and Like

- Set of three: Advanced Clinicals Complete Skin Care Set with Anti-Aging Retinol Serum; Plumping Collagen Serum; and Vitamin C Serum
- Radha Beauty Hyaluronic Acid Serum with Vitamin C, Vitamin E, Green Tea and Jojoba Oil
- Radha Miracle Retinol Moisturizer
- Pure Body Naturals Organic Shea Butter & Retinol Night Cream Moisturizer

Let me interject that I buy most of my creams and beauty products on Amazon because it is convenient and saves time shopping; plus, I can compare products. I always read the customer reviews and rely on them only if there are a substantial number of verified positive purchases, and I also read the questions and answers section.

I might as well confess that I am not a person that is patient or practices "moderation." Having said that, I sometimes layer several creams on my face before I put on makeup. I don't know if this overkill increases the results or just makes me happy. Whatever—I have had significant changes in the youthfulness of my face!

Dry Brushing Skin

(Created by Dr. Paavo Airola over 30 years ago) https://naturalhealthtechniques. com/healingtechniquesdry_brushing_technique/

Dry Brushing provides a gentle internal massage and particularly deals with detoxification of the skin.

Benefits of Dry Brushing

- Removes cellulite
- Cleanses the lymphatic system
- Removes dead skin layers
- Strengthens the immune system
- Stimulates the hormone and oil-producing glands
- Tightens the skin preventing premature aging

- Tones the muscles

- Stimulates circulation

- Improves the function of the nervous system

- Helps digestion

How to Dry Brush

- Use a soft natural fiber brush with a long handle, loofah, or a rough towel.

- Brush prior to bathing or showering.

- Begin with your feet and brush vigorously in circular motions.

- Continue brushing up your legs.

- Proceed to your hands and arms.

- Brush your entire back and abdomen area, shoulders, and neck.

- Use circular counter-clockwise strokes on the abdomen.

- Lightly brush the breasts.

- Brush upwards on the back and down from the neck. Better yet, have a friend, spouse or family member brush your back.

Oil Up

- After Dry Brushing, I slather Green Coffee Bean Oil, Avocado Oil, Macadamia Oil, or Thermo-Firming Cream and Genes Vitamin E Crème all over my body before taking a shower and allow it to absorb into my skin from the heat of the water. Additionally, I put more on my arms when

I get out of the shower while my body is still warm. This has worked better than any other techniques I've used to reduce crepiness and the products are relatively inexpensive. My arms are decidedly improved but aren't yet perfect, and I've used it for less than a month at this writing.

Specific Skin Problems

Generally skin problems are symptoms of something that needs fixing internally; therefore, the below remedies for "fixing" skin problems should be preceded by cleaning up your diet by eating only natural, healthy foods (yes, again).

Crepey Skin

I've used many popular body lotions and creams to get rid of the dryness and crepiness on my arms but have been disappointed in the results or, in fact, no results. As a caveat, I will say that most of the products I've used and discontinued have made my skin itch, so they probably have an ingredient to which I am allergic, such as quaternium, polyquaternium, and other chemicals.

Recently I ordered **Advanced Clinicals' "Green Coffee Bean Oil"** to test on my skin. The jar advertises that it is "for tummy, hips, upper arms, and body" and "reduces the appearance of cellulite [and] gives cellulite-prone skin a more toned and tightened look, with invigorating tea extract, paraben-free." Big promises. It has worked somewhat for me.

I also ordered **"Thermo-Firming Cream"** and **"Genes Vitamin E Crème, Swiss Collagen Complex for Dry and Sensitive Skin."** It contains vitamins E, A & D plus Panthenol and Allantoin. It also has improved my crepey skin.

These heavy creams seem to produce more results for me than lotions, creams, or any other products for crepey skin with the exception of **FineVine Organic Almond Oil.**

Skin Tags

- **Oregano oil.** A powerful antiseptic and antispasmodic to help the skin tag dry on its own. For best results, apply 5–6 drops of oregano oil to the tag three times a day with changes occurring in about a month.

- **Castor oil and baking soda.** Mix the two ingredients to make a thick paste. Dip a cotton swab in the paste and dab it on the skin tag.

- **Lemon juice.** The acid in lemon juice works wonders on skin tags. Lemon juice is not only acidic but also a powerful antiseptic.

Age Spots

- **Onion and apple cider vinegar.** Apply a mixture made from equal parts onion juice and apple cider vinegar directly to the age spot to help remove the blemish.

- **Horseradish and milk.** Soak raw horseradish in a bowl of milk for 20–30 minutes. Apply the treated milk to the age spots. The antioxidants and volatile compounds will help the age spots fade and eventually disappear.

- **Buttermilk and tomato.** This odd combination of ingredients is an effective natural remedy for age spots. Both the tomato and buttermilk contain potent acids.

Moles

- **Cumin.** Make a paste of ground cumin and water, and apply it to your moles over a period of three weeks.

- **Flaxseeds and honey**. Flaxseed oil helps to remove moles naturally, while honey aids in preventing secondary infection and scaring. Apply, leave on an hour, and then wash with lukewarm water.

Warts

- **Apple Cider Vinegar.** Apply apple cider vinegar directly to the wart once a day. The best way is to soak a cotton ball in the vinegar and then fix it over the wart using a band-aid.

- **Pineapple juice.** Soaking your warts in pineapple juice exposes it to acids which eat away at the wart.

Blackheads

- **Baking soda.** As an antiseptic, baking soda cleans your skin, helps to neutralize the pH levels, and encourages your skin to produce less oil thereby reducing blackheads.

- **Oatmeal.** This breakfast food also makes a great cleanser, working to loosen up the debris stuck in your pores and eliminate blackheads.

- **Lemon juice.** Lemon Juice contains alpha-hydroxy acid (AHA), citric acid, which works to remove dead skin and loosen clogged pores.

Caring for your skin is not optional if you aspire to being a senior beauty!!!

Makeup

Up front, let me be clear, I will not presume to give you advice on what makeup to use, how to apply it, and what looks best on you. I don't know! However, I will give you some tips I have learned and sites that will give instructions on makeup for mature ladies. Plus, I encourage you to get an expert's one-time guidance on how to look younger with makeup. Warning, before going to an "expert," thoroughly check them out on the internet, particularly the "complaints" listed about them.

Margianna's Tips

- Shape your face with your hair; e.g., my face is wide at the temples so I make sure my hair covers this area; if you have a high forehead, partial bangs that will lower your forehead may be in order.

- First of all, create a blank canvas on your face before applying makeup. By that I mean use cream, primer, concealer, and foundation to hide any imperfections you have on your face such as under-eye dark circles and hollows, dark spots, wrinkles and any other thing that is hiding your facial beauty. After this is done, it will appear as if you do not have on makeup, just have a perfect complexion. I use several Neutrogena products because they are good products and because I'm not allergic to them. Different skin types require different kinds of products and, for me, I have to be careful that the makeup I use doesn't produce an allergic reaction (swollen eyes or face, itching, rash, redness, etc.).

- Prevent an "old lady" look by making sure you put on makeup under bright lights—no bright red rosy cheeks, raccoon eyes, red lips, etc. Most of the time, I recheck my makeup once I get in the car and have the advantage of the sun's light to clearly see what others are seeing when they look at me.

More Information on Makeup

Sixty & Me (http://sixtyandme.com/14-exclusive-makeup-tips-for-older-women-from-a-professional-makeup-artist/)

- Shape Natural Brows: brush your eyebrows down, draw a light line along the top of the brow line and then brush the brows up again.

- Eye Shadow: do not extend color beyond the end of the eye because this can make your face look tired and accentuates jowls. [Note: I extend eye pencil and/or eye shadow beyond the eye in an upward sweep from the end of the eye. This makes my eyes look larger and more dramatic without making my face look tired and unattractive.]

- Mascara: avoid lengthening and curling mascaras, and choose a thickening formula to make lashes look full and lush. [Note: This is your preference. I like full and long!]

- Use eyeliner and mascara in navy blue to make eyes look whiter. [Note: Use if navy blue is one of your preferred colors].

- Apply cream blush with a brush to the apple of the cheek. Smile to find the right spot. This will emphasize eyes and not wrinkles.

- Make lips voluptuous by placing highlighter above your lips.

Many more sites for makeup for senior women can be found by entering an internet search for "Makeup for Older Women."

SMILE!!!

Shinier, Thicker, Healthier Hair

As a heads up, **Dr. Al Sears in Ageless Beauty Secrets** says that Rogaine, a popular treatment for hair loss, is dangerous. It can have side effects like dizziness, fainting, and difficulty breathing. The good news is there are natural ways to maintain thick, healthy hair.

The ancient Indian spice known as fenugreek (Trigonella foenum-graecum) can help build thicker hair in both men and women because it contains vitamin B3, or Niacin, which is a vasodilator that stimulates blood flow to the hair follicles. An easy way to consume ground fenugreek is by adding it to food (stir-fries, soups, smoothies).

Other ways to increase the thickness, luster, and health of hair

- **Stimulate your scalp** with fenugreek.
- **Enhance thickness** by applying ginseng to make each strand thick and strong.
- **Feed the hair** with amino acids, the building blocks of hair structure.
- **Ingest the nutrients**, particularly B-vitamins, that are essential to growing healthy hair and nails.

- **Promote that shine** - Hydrolyzed soy protein can give you shinier, thicker hair that stays moisturized. (I use Hawaiian Silky, recommended by my hairdresser, for a leave-in conditioner.)

Dr. Josh Axe – *a wealth of information and natural remedies can be found on Dr. Axe's website* (https://draxe.com/)

Supplements to Encourage Hair Health (Dr. Axe)

1. Fish Oil – nourishes the hair; supports hair thickening; reduces inflammation

2. Zinc – benefits hair follicle health

3. B-Complex – Biotin rebuilds hair cuticle, B5 supports the adrenal glands that stimulate hair growth

4. Iron – prevents hair loss

5. Vitamin C – fights free radical damage

6. Vitamin D – helps prevent damage to hair follicles

Harmful Shampoo Ingredients

(https://www.nutrafol.com/blog/15-shampoo-ingredients-to-avoid/)

1. Ammonium Lauryl Sulfate or Sodium Laureth Sulfate (SLES)

2. Sodium Lauryl Sulfate (SLS)

3. Parabens

4. Sodium Chloride

5. Polyethylene Glycols (PEG)

6. Diethanolamine (DEA)

7. Triethanolamine (TEA)

8. Formaldehyde

9. Alcohol

10. Synthetic Fragrances

11. Synthetic Colors

12. Dimethicone

13. Cocamidopropyl Betaine

14. Triclosan

15. Retinyl Palmitate

Harmless Shampoo Ingredients

The list of shampoo ingredients that are harmful is extensive, and it can be difficult to keep track of all of them. However, there are plenty of brands that use only natural and organic ingredients, and you can even make your own homemade hair treatments using things from your kitchen.

> You can find many recipes for homemade masks for different hair problems at https://www.diyncrafts.com/34150/beauty/15-natural-homemade-hair-masks-give-healthy-beautiful-hair.

Better than Hair Masks

The best tip to maintain a healthy head of hair is to simply eat and live well. If you are stressed for a period of time or feel that you need an extra boost, there are many natural hair supplements to take (with your doctor's approval). After taking **Life Code's Stem Cell** for a couple of months, new hair appeared around my temples, even though I didn't take it for that purpose. The new hair growth continued when I switched to taking **Life Code's Telomax** instead of Stem Cell. Check out their site for good information and researched and tested supplements that I trust. (https://www.lifecoderx.com/)

Hair Shape and Style

My changing look!

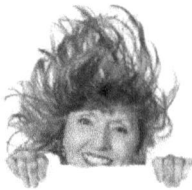

Bad Hair Day

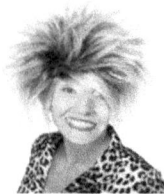

Wild & Wooly

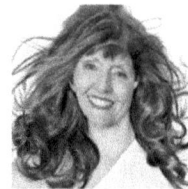

Glamorous
(I wish!)

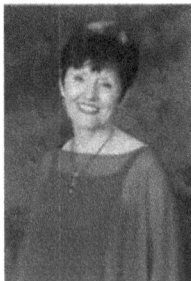

The Real Me
(15 years ago)

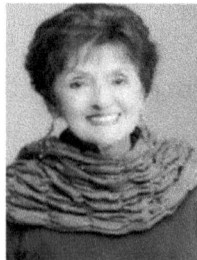

The Real Me
(81 years old)

Have fun virtually trying on hundreds of hairstyles and discover information to enhance your look at https://www.thehairstyler.com/face-shape-quiz.

Go to https://www.thehairstyler.com/ (https://www.thehairstyler.com/virtual-hairstyler).

Mature Women's Stylish Hair

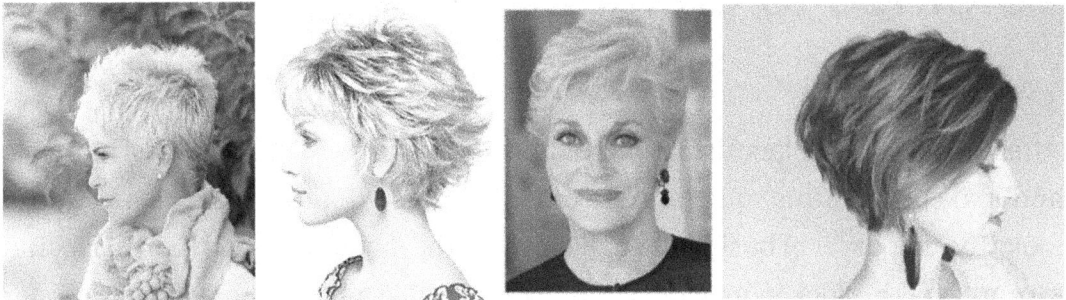

The secret to maintaining or achieving beautiful hair is to be healthy in body, mind, and spirit! Commit to incorporating supportive lifestyle habits, including eating a clean diet, exercising, getting sufficient sleep, and having a positive outlook. (Are you tired of hearing this? Well, it's that important!)

Continue reading to further improve your youthful look by choosing clothes, colors and styles, which enhance your complexion and overall appearance.

Look Your Best:
Clothes to Enhance Your Appearance

After preparing your face using creams and fillers and choosing your best hairstyle and makeup, it's time to determine other ways to enhance or create a youthful look. The first order of business is to determine the look you want to portray … find examples of this look in magazines or on the internet and personalize this look for yourself. Your personality is often a good indicator of what type of style suits you best. For example, a woman who is soft-spoken and likes to daydream typically gravitates toward frilly pieces like lace and ruffles. A culture-loving person tends to dress more urban and sporty than most fashionistas.

> Check out Jennifer Baumgartner's book, *You Are What You Wear: What Your Clothes Reveal About You,* to help you correctly portray your identity.

Also, to help you determine your style, go to https://www.proprofs.com/quiz-school/story.php?title=whats-your-personal-fashion-style and take the quiz. I did and the quiz was correct if limited to only the categories listed. The results said I like classic clothes and that is true, but I also like elegant clothes which were not a choice!

Check out the following styles of clothes. Frankly, various designers and fashion stores each have their own interpretation of styles. Take in all the information, decide what look makes you happy and feel good, and go with that.

Clothes Styles

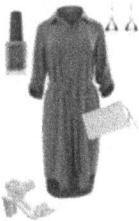 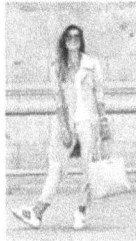 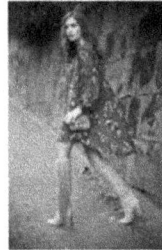 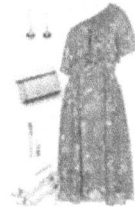

| Classic | Relaxed | Expressive | Romantic |

- **Classic**: Timeless pieces and structured fits attract the classic personality. The classic avoids fussy prints, trends, and attention-seeking pieces. She looks to style icons like Grace Kelly, Jackie O, and Kate Middleton for inspiration. The classic is all about tweeds, blazers, crisp white blouses, pencil skirts, dark denim, pearls, ballet flats, and menswear-inspired outerwear. She's always prepared for every occasion.

- **Relaxed**: Comfort is number one for the relaxed personality. But, the relaxed fashion personality knows that being comfortable doesn't mean looking like a slob! Relaxed personalities know how to look effortlessly cool in cotton shirts, neutral colors, slouchy knits, drop-waist dresses, loose trousers, chambrays, boyfriend jeans, maxi skirts, and chic sneakers.

- **Expressive**: The expressive fashion personality chooses bold articles of clothing and often considers fashion an art form. Every day is a chance to create a unique masterpiece! Not afraid to try trends or stand out in a crowd, expressives gravitate toward bright colors, funky patterns, and chunky jewelry.

- **Romantic:** Those with a romantic personality will gravitate toward twirling midi skirts, floral patterns, blushing pinks, silk blouses, pearls, and antique jewelry. The romantic loves to enhance her natural beauty by incorporating feminine details and flattering fits. She isn't just frills and bows—her personality is expressed through many different styles and finds inspiration from vintage Hollywood, the Victorian Era, the country, 18th-century France (a la Marie Antoinette), and many more.

Other styles identified by designers include: Trendy, Casual, Elegant, Exotic, Vibrant, Sexy, Preppy, Elegant, Bohemian, Girly, Cowgirl, Girl Next Door, Punk, Artsy, Businesswoman, Tomboy, Gothic, Rocker, 50s, 70s and Sporty.

Colors to Enhance Your Look

After determining your style, the next step is to discover the colors that enhance your look! That is, the colors that highlight your complexion and hair while helping to hide imperfections. Did you know that wearing an unflattering color for your complexion emphasizes and draws attention to your imperfections, including wrinkles, dark circles under the eyes, dark skin spots, sallow and sagging skin, and moles and skin tags? No one I know has the goal to wear an unflattering color to show off these unattractive features!

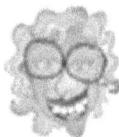

Many years ago I went to a trained consultant (colormebeautiful.com) who determined the colors that showed off my face to its best advantage. When I went back to work with a different color scheme and more flattering makeup, the young doctors for whom I worked had one word … "sultry." I was excited!!! Let me hasten to add that that's not the word I would covet at my current age—words like "younger" or "more vibrant" now make me smile!

I recommend engaging a color consultant to get an expert opinion on your best colors or purchase the **Color Me Beautiful: 4 Seasons of Color, Makeup, and Style** *book to enhance your knowledge and, as the cover says: reinvent yourself.*

Also, have a party!!! Invite several interested friends over and, one by one, help each other determine your best colors. Be sure to remove all makeup and cover hair to judge the best color scheme for your complexion.

You may have been "colored" when you were younger, but it is wise to have your colors analyzed again after you reach 50. In the *Color Me Beautiful* book, I learned that a person's best colors can change as she gets older. This explained why I was identified as an "Autumn" when I was in my 20s and 30s and later identified as a "Winter" in my 50s.

The following information is not mine but is borrowed from the Color Me Beautiful book as well as being readily available on the internet with a savvy search. It will give you clues for deciding if you are a "warm" or "cool" system.

Determine Your Best Colors

Warm or Cool

Your current hair color, not your hair color as a child, is the most important characteristic in determining if you fit into the warm or cool color pattern. Clues are as follows:

Warm

- Hair has golden or red hues
  - Red, copper, or auburn
  - Golden blonde
  - Brown with golden or red highlights (chestnut brown)
  - Gold gray

- Eye color when looking in mirror with natural lighting
  - Gold or brown flecks in eyes
  - Dark brown, hazel, amber brown, or red-brown
  - Blue eyes with brown flecks
  - Green, aqua or turquoise, or olive green

- Complexion
  - Peachy or ivory
  - Golden beige or golden bronze
  - Caramel, latte, maple or dark coppery beige
  - Ruddiness appears most often in warm skin tones
  - Freckles

Cool

o Hair has no red or gold highlights

- Platinum blonde
- Jet-black, off-black, blue-black
- Ash brown
- Ash blonde
- Pearl gray, salt and pepper
- Silver

o Eyes have no golden tones

- Deep black
- Black brown
- Charcoal
- Blue eyes with white, gray, or blue tones

o Complexion

- Porcelain white
- Mahogany (medium brown with reddish-brown cast — found among those from African and Native American descent)
- Freckles are rosy or charcoal gray
- Black, olive and beige skin tones can be cool if they have blue, red or pink undertones
- Wrists veins are blue

Now that you have completed the most difficult step in color analysis, which is, deciding if you are "warm" or "cool," the next step is to subdivide these categories into "seasons" to fine tune your best colors even more. The cool seasons are Summer and Winter, and the warm seasons are Autumn and Spring. Following are characteristics of each of the seasons.

Four Seasons

Autumn

Warm and deep – among notable autumns are Gloria Estefan, Jennifer Lopez, Mariah Carey, and Serena Williams

- o Hair

  - Bright copper red, rich golden red
  - Deep chestnut brown, golden brown, dark warm brown, light, medium or dark ash brown with ash highlights
  - Blonde
  - Cover gray with warm blonde or gold highlights

- o Skin – golden undertones that will appear more orange than blue

  - Ivory
  - Peach
  - Golden beige
  - Bronze
  - Caramel, maple or latte to golden brown
  - Ruddy skin
  - Many Native Americans, Latinas, Asians, Africans, Middle Eastern and Mediterraneans are autumn

- o Eyes - golden warmth in the iris – majority will have brown, warm hazel with golden brown or green gold tones or green eyes

  - Dark brown, golden brown, indefinite brownish
  - Green, indefinite greenish
  - Amber

- o Complimentary Colors

  - Ivory, cream
  - Taupe, terra cotta, rust

- Turquoise, medium aqua
- Golden or dark Brown, bronze
- Salmon, coral, deep peach, tomato red
- Olive, moss, lime
- Periwinkle, purple
- Gold

Spring

Warm and light – among notable springs are Diane Sawyer, Ellen DeGeneres, Gwyneth Paltrow

o Hair

- Golden, strawberry, or beige blonde
- Copper, caramel
- Champagne

o Skin – warm or golden undertones – always a delicate look

- Creamy ivory
- Peach, peach beige
- Golden beige
- May have sprinkle of golden or light blonde freckles or ruddy complexion
- Typically light skinned
- Ruddy skin

o Eyes - springs do not have deep brown eyes

- Blue
- Green
- Aqua
- Warm amber, warm hazel with golden brown or green gold tones, blue green, topaz, caramel, or turquoise

- Complementary Colors
  - Ivory, cream, taupe, camel
  - Light or clear aqua, powder blue
  - Coffee or golden brown, bronze
  - Salmon, peach, clear red
  - Lime, mint, yellow green
  - Bright periwinkle, purple
  - Bright golden yellow, gold

Winter

Cool and deep colors – among notable winters are Barbara Bush, Halle Berry, Connie Chung

- Hair - no red or gold highlights
  - Gray
  - Jet black, blue-black, brown-black
  - Medium to dark brown with ash, silver, white and salt and pepper highlights

- Eyes - deep, dark eye color
  - Black, black brown
  - Charcoal, gray-blue, or gray-green
  - Red brown to cool hazel with blue or green

- Skin
  - Porcelain white
  - Beige, rosy beige, and cool beige
  - Mahogany
  - Black, olive and beige skin tones can be cool if they have blue, red, or pink undertones

- Many Africans, Asians, Native Americans, Latinas, and Middle Eastern people are Winters
- Winter shades will brighten the whites of your eyes

o Some of the winter colors – deep and bright cool colors

- White, black, gray
- Hot pink, fuchsia, cranberry, burgundy
- Emerald green, turquoise, teal
- True blue, royal blue
- Bright and deep periwinkle, purple, violet

Summer

Cool and pastel colors – among notable summers are Queen Elizabeth, Jennifer Aniston, and Diane Keaton

o Hair

- Gray
- Brown – light, medium, or dark ash brown with ash highlights
- Blonde

o Skin – pink rose or blue skin undertones

- Lightest porcelain
- Pale, neutral, cool or rose beige
- Freckles are rare but are charcoal gray or rosy
- Pink skin or cheeks

o Eyes - no brown-eyed summers

- Blue or green with white flecks, gray-blue aqua, blue green, blue gray
- Gray, grayish
- Cool hazel with blue or green

- ○ Colors
    - ▪ Soft white
    - ▪ Charcoal
    - ▪ Taupe
    - ▪ Gray-blue, powder blue, medium aqua
    - ▪ Pink, rose, raspberry, lavender, amethyst, purple
    - ▪ Light lemon yellow
    - ▪ Light teal, emerald turquoise, blue green
    - ▪ Silver

Body Shapes

The clothes you choose should enhance your body type, meaning they highlight good parts and camouflage imperfections. Check out the following basic types:

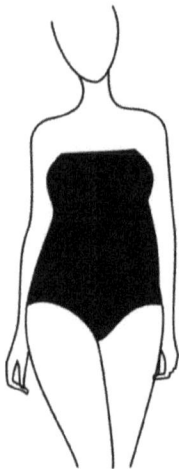 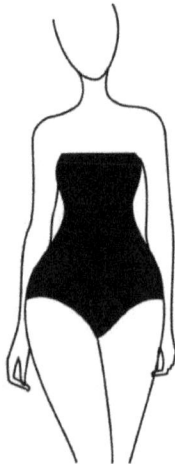 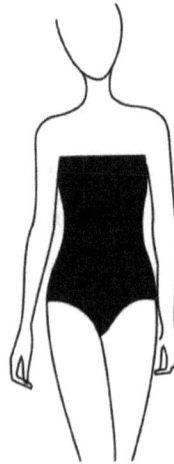 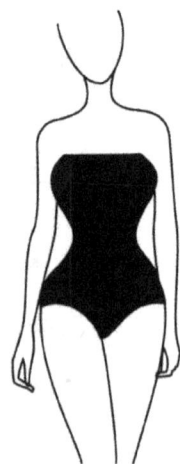

APPLE   **PEAR**   **RECTANGLE**   **HOURGLASS**

1. **Apple body type.** "Top-heavy" type includes approximately 14 percent of women; the bust is three or more inches bigger than the hips. https://www.joyofclothes.com/style-advice/shape-guides/the-apple.php

   - Slim limbs, specifically the arms, and wide shoulders are a typical characteristic of this body type.

   - Weight is concentrated around midsection and chest, giving the appearance of a bigger bust and protruding stomach at times.

   - Just below the midsection, the waistline can have a little definition, thus giving rise to the "top-heavy" description of this body type.

   - Though your top may be on the heavier side, your legs will be slimmer.

2. **Pear body type.** "Bottom-heavy" (or triangle) types are about 20 percent of women. Pears have hips significantly larger than bust. https://shopyourshape.com/body-shapes/pear-shaped-body/

   - Your lower body: hips, thighs, and sometimes your behind are more noticeable.

   - Shoulders are narrow and sloping.

   - "Curvaceous" body with legs that are wider, muscular, and fuller compared to the rest of your body.

3. **Straight/rectangular body type.** About 46 percent of women are this shape where the waist is about the same size as hips and bust. https://www.joyofclothes.com/style-advice/shape-guides/the-lean-column.php

   - Standing up straight, you should not notice any significant curves around the waist area.

- Your rib cage will define most of your shape, as there will be no waist definition to add curves.

- Despite being rectangular, you may still have a curvy bottom (similar to a pear bottom), or a wide chest with a little bit of extra weight around the midriff.

4. **Hourglass body type.** This is the least common with only 8 percent of women having this body type. The hip and bust measurements are usually equal, with a narrow waist. https://www.joyofclothes.com/style-advice/shape-guides/the-full-hourglass.php

- Unlike other body shapes, the hourglass figure has a significantly defined waist.

- Looking in the mirror, your hip line and bust line are the same width.

- You can still have an hourglass body even when: slightly fleshy upper arms, wider looking shoulders, and a slightly fuller bottom.

In which category do you fit?
Apple_____Pear_____Straight/Rectangular_____Hourglass_____

Dress for Your Body Type

1. **Apple** — direct attention away from your midriff and wear clothes to accentuate other parts.

- Keep details on the top and lower third of your body. With this body type, it is easy to wear shirts, blouses or dresses with slight V-necks.

- Draw attention away from your waist and shoulders/arms (wear long sleeves), and draw attention to your bust and neck, such as with v-necklines.

- Choose flared pants over straight-leg or skinny pants to help balance out wide shoulders and/or a heavy upper body. Wear bottoms just below your hipbone to draw attention away from your midriff.

- Avoid dresses and belts that pinch at your waist. This will most likely accentuate curves that you may not wish to show off.

2. **Pear** — wear anything that adds to your shoulder and bust area. Keep attention to your upper body by minimizing the lower half.

   - Balance your top with your bottom. Try to wear tops that accentuate your shoulders a bit more.

   - Avoid pants or tights that narrow your legs.

   - Wear a bra that adds to or enhances your bust.

   - Wear straight-leg or slightly flared pants with heels. Skinny pants that hug your ankles can make your lower body take on the appearance of an upside-down triangle.

3. **Straight or rectangular** — With this body type, you may have a long, thin body that tends to lack curves. It is sometimes referred to as a "boyish" profile.

   - If you have this body type, you can "pinch" in your waist to exaggerate curves. For example, add a belt to your dress.

   - Go for ruffles and frills to add texture, volume, and femininity to your figure.

- Steer clear of menswear-style clothing. For example, dressing in baggy jeans and track clothes will make you look like "one of the boys" but not a potential girlfriend.

- Stock up on miniskirts and bright tights to make the most of your great legs. They will also add more shape to a straight body.

- Use shapewear — a rectangular body type benefits from shaping undergarments. For example, a bra that adds a cup size will balance out your angular features.

4. **Hourglass** — avoid anything that makes you look "boxy"! You have admirable curves, so embrace them.

- Use your waist as the focal point when dressing. Wear snug clothes and accessories around the thinnest part of your waist that will make your curves stand out even more.

- Dress to flatter your beautiful curves by following your body's outline. Tailored clothing is usually more flattering.

- Balance your top and bottom while accentuating your waist.

- Shape your bust. If you have an hourglass shape, you probably have plenty of bust; your main concern should be to wear a supportive bra so that your chest looks perky, not droopy and saggy.

- Embrace V-neck dresses and tops.

Shopping Guidelines

It doesn't pay financially to go shopping when it is necessary for you to buy an outfit for a special event. You are making a decision to pay top dollar! Instead, stop in your favorite outlet store or mall store that is having a sale and look for clothes you will need in the future. I frequently visit discount stores such as Ross, Burlington, and TJ Maxx, quickly look at what they offer, and either buy an item at a great price or leave the store quickly. Also, I have purchased many casual and dressy tops at Sam's Club for under $10.

> When my sister and I were teenagers, we learned to love bargains like our mother. Finally, my dad observed our bargain-buying sprees and said, "If you buy any more bargains, we're going to the poorhouse!" (We continued our buying habits and, fortunately, never went to the "poorhouse.")

You might have guessed I do not like shopping; however, I do like buying. I will only go in a mall if I can enter a store from an outside entrance, so I can quickly look and leave. The chemicals on clothes trigger my allergies to the point that I have difficulty thinking, particularly when making a decision to buy or leave.

> *Hint: I learned that if I go into department stores the week **after** the "After Christmas Sales," I find great bargains. For instance, I bought two suits at a two-for-one sale at Macy's, one a Jones of New York that was originally priced at $325 and the other a Kasper that originally was priced at $250; I purchased them both for $75! Oh, happy day—and I didn't go to the "poor house."*

To conserve time, scan the stores clothing racks quickly by doing the following:

1. Find your size.

2. Quickly look for your colors and only look at those that are your colors—don't waste your time looking at something you are not going to (or shouldn't) buy.

3. Look at the style to see if it will enhance your look and body shape (for example, if a blouse is to be tucked in, I immediately dismiss it because I am short-waisted).

4. Check the price. As previously stated, I only go for the bargains!

Now that you are gorgeous, it's time to add a few "odds and ends" and gourmet cooking skills to your knowledge. In the following chapter is a section with wonderful recipes shared by my friend who is an incredible cook. Following that chapter, you'll get beneficial tips (Odds and Ends) that will save you time and trouble discovering for yourself.

Section Four
~

Yummy Foods and Beneficial Spices: Eat to Stay Young and Healthy

Eating a healthy diet does not have to be boring or repetitive. While you may think making the change to a natural, clean way of eating leaves you with limited choices; in reality, there is an overwhelming number of delicious, healthy choices available. The best diet consists of fresh, unprocessed foods with ingredients you can recognize. With that said, following are delicious foods made from natural ingredients.

But, before I share the recipes, let me introduce you to someone I'm blessed to know, my friend Layla Lusty. Layla and I first met and decided to room together over thirty-one years ago. I watched with fascination at how vivacious and fun-loving Layla was and truthfully wanted to be like her.

All these many years, we have belonged to the same spiritual group, each of us has grown, and our lives changed, (she married) but we've remained friends. However, things were a bit dicey when we first became roommates. I prepared my favorite Southern dish of rice and black-eyed peas with onions, salt, and pepper, then left it to simmer on the stovetop. Looking forward to this wonderful meal, I served myself a big bowl and was shocked with the first mouthful; I couldn't believe what had happened to my favorite dish. It had a strange, exotic taste that was not to my liking. Layla had "improved" it. It was not my Southern delicacy anymore but a "Mediterranean delight." In no uncertain terms, I told Layla, "Don't ever mess with my black-eyed peas again!" And we're still friends!

Why am I telling you about Layla? Because she is a gourmet cook and serves delicious foods at the many gatherings we share. She is also the creator of the Facebook group Chocolate Lovers Society that has over 7,000 members. Her foods are always made from original, creative recipes and natural ingredients, taste special, and are beautifully presented.

When seeing Layla's beautiful food, I am reminded of what my former son-in-law, a chef, always said: "Presentation is everything."

Enough with the introduction and onto the important information. I asked Layla to give the readers of my book a gift of some of her recipes and she agreed. Without further ado, following are several of Layla's delicious recipes and their photographs, followed by some of my favorite recipes.

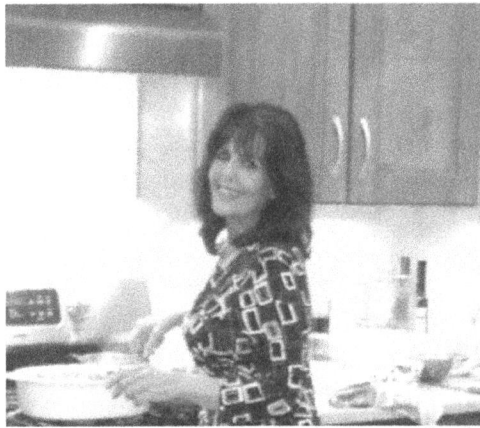

Layla

Recipes From the Kitchen of Layla

Charred Corn, Black Beans, and Avocado Salad

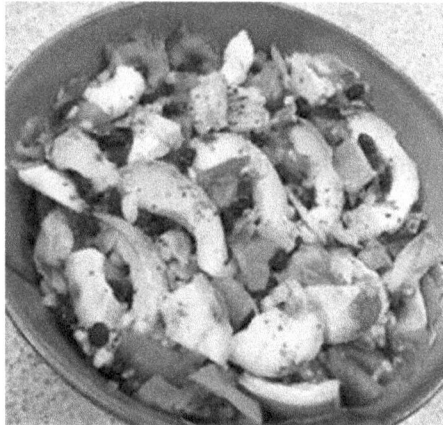

Mixed Salad Greens

One ear of corn, steamed then charred over a hot iron grill

1 cup black beans

2 medium tomatoes

1/2 medium red onion, thinly sliced

2 medium avocados

Balsamic Vinaigrette:

1/2 cup balsamic vinegar

1 tablespoon Dijon mustard

1 garlic clove, minced or crushed

1/2 cup olive oil

Salt and pepper

In a bowl, mix the balsamic vinegar, mustard, and garlic. Add the olive oil slowly, whisking constantly. Season with salt and pepper. Set aside.

Salad:

Place the mixed green corn, beans, tomatoes, and onions in a salad bowl. Toss in half the balsamic vinaigrette. Top with slices of avocado. Sprinkle the rest of the balsamic vinaigrette over everything. Serve as a side or main dish with warm baguette.

Tabbouleh

1/2 cup bulgur or couscous

3 tomatoes, seeded and finely chopped

2 cucumbers, finely chopped

3 green onions or 1/2 red onion, finely chopped

2 cups fresh parsley, finely chopped

1/2 cup fresh mint leaves, finely chopped

1 teaspoons salt

1/2 cup lemon juice

2/3 cup olive oil

1/2 teaspoon allspice or cumin powder

A sprinkle of black pepper

1 teaspoon maple syrup or honey

1. Place the bulgur in bowl and cover with 1 cup boiling water. Soak for 30 minutes; drain and squeeze out excess water. You can use couscous same way, but soak only 5 minutes or so. I love it with couscous.

2. In a mixing bowl, combine the bulgur or couscous, tomatoes, cucumbers, onions, parsley, and mint. Mix together and add salt, pepper, allspice, lemon juice, olive oil, and maple syrup.

3. Toss and serve or refrigerate for 1 hour or more before serving. Toss again prior to serving.

Roasted Beets, Caramelized Pear and Blue Cheese Salad

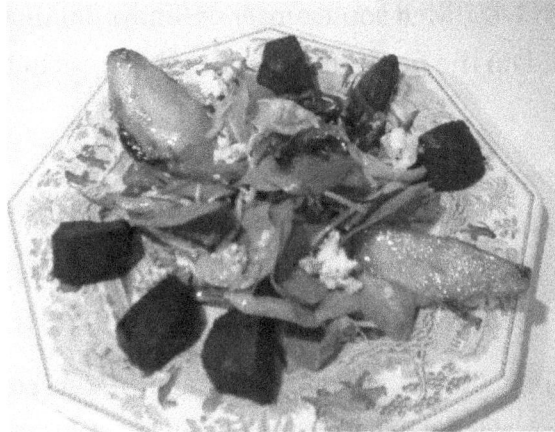

3 medium beets

3 ripe pears

1 bunch watercress

1/2 cup brown sugar

2 tablespoons butter or Smart Balance

1 cup crumbled Gorgonzola or blue cheese

1/2 cup balsamic vinaigrette (recipe found in Charred Corn, Black Beans, and Avocado Salad recipe on page 144)

1. Preheat the oven to 380 degrees F.

2. Wash the beets thoroughly, leaving the skins on, then remove the greens and save them for other dishes. Place the beets in a roasting pan, and toss with 2 tablespoons of olive oil. If you wish to peel the beets, it is easier to do so once they have been roasted.

3. Cover and bake for 45 to 60 minutes, or until a knife can slide easily through the largest beet.

4. When the roasted beets are done, let cool, then peel them by rubbing the skin with your fingers or peel with a knife. Cut off the tops and bottoms of beets.

5. Cut the pears into 1/8's. Melt some butter or Smart Balance in a pot but do not let brown or boil. Dip the pears in the butter then toss in brown sugar to coat all sides.

6. Heat a roasting pan in the oven till very hot. Take out and place the coated pears on it and return to the 380 degree oven. Cook approximately 5 minutes while checking often, and turn over when the underside is caramelized. Let cool.

7. Toss the watercress in the vinaigrette. Place in the center of each plate. Surround with the roasted beets and caramelized pears.

8. Sprinkle with crumbled blue or Gorgonzola cheese and serve.

Avocado & Tomato Salad

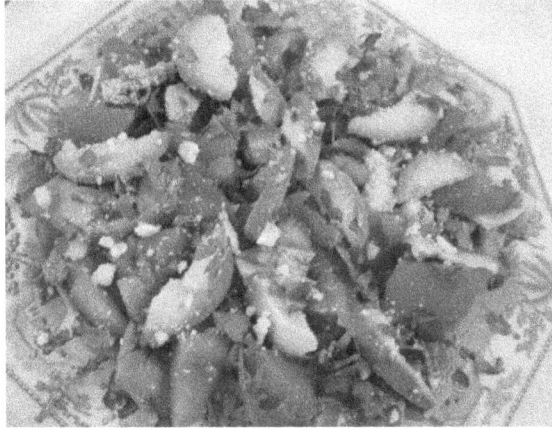

2 avocados
2 large tomatoes
Mixed salad greens or 1 bunch water cress
1 cup crumbled Gorgonzola, blue, or feta cheese
1 cup vinaigrette
Salt & pepper

1. Wash and dry the greens or watercress and toss with 1/2 the vinaigrette. Arrange evenly on a large serving platter.

2. Slice the tomatoes into quarters and arrange over the greens. Sprinkle lightly with salt and pepper.

3. Peel and slice the avocados in lengthwise slices and arrange over the tomatoes.

4. Sprinkle the remaining vinaigrette over everything, then add the crumbled cheese evenly over the salad.

Yummers!

Carrot Coriander Soup

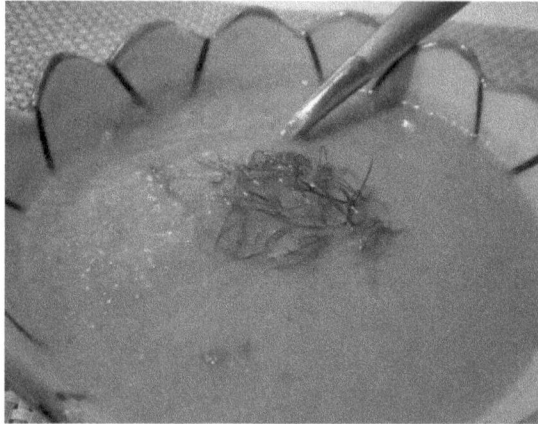

1 onion, medium diced

5 large carrots, medium diced

1 sweet potato, medium diced

1 teaspoon crushed fresh garlic

salt & pepper

1 teaspoon coriander seeds, roughly ground

Pinch of dry thyme

1 teaspoon curry powder

A handful of fresh cilantro, chopped

3 cups chicken or vegetable broth

1/2 lime

Zest from 1/2 lime

1 teaspoon maple syrup or honey

1. Sauté 1 onion, 5 large carrots, 1 sweet potato, all medium diced.

2. Add a teaspoon of fresh crushed garlic, salt & pepper, 1 teaspoon of roughly ground coriander seeds, a pinch of dry thyme, 1 teaspoon curry powder, chopped fresh cilantro. Sauté a little longer.

3. Add chicken or vegetable broth.

4. Bring to boil then simmer for about 25 minutes till veggies are very tender.

5. Squeeze 1/2 a lime, and zest of 1/2 lime, 1 teaspoon maple syrup or honey.

6. Put everything in the food processor or use the hand-held blender and blend together till smooth.

Delicious and nutritious!

Chocolate Guinness Pudding

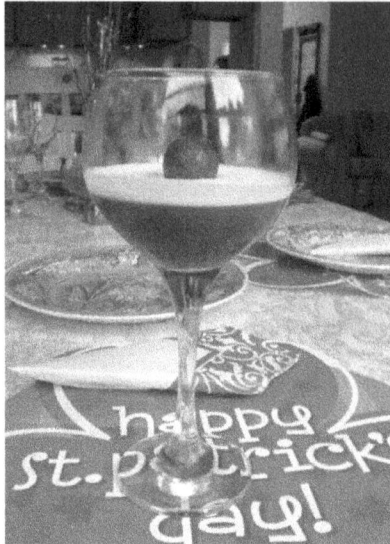

3 eggs

1/3 cup all-purpose flour

1/2 cup brown sugar

1 cup Guinness beer

1 cup chocolate almond milk

1/2 teaspoon vanilla extract

1-1/2 cups dark or semisweet chocolate chips

1 cup whipped cream

Pinch salt

1. Combine eggs, sugar, salt and flour in a mixing bowl. Whisk till smooth.

2. Place a saucepan over medium heat, pour in the chocolate almond milk and the Guinness beer. Heat until almost boiling. Remove from heat.

3. Slowly pour the Guinness mixture into the egg mixture, whisking constantly until well combined.

4. Pour the mixture back into the saucepan and bring to boil. Reduce the heat and simmer gently for about 15 minutes or till the pudding is thick and bubbly. Remove from heat.

5. Stir in the chocolate chips and vanilla till melted. Pour pudding into four large wine glasses or four medium tumblers or the serving dishes of your choice. Cover with plastic wrap; refrigerate till cold and set.

6. Top pudding with whipped cream and serve. May the Guinness rise up to meet you!

Thanks to Layla for the wonderful recipes and photographs.

(Layla, can we persuade you to publish a cook book?)

Herbs and Spices for a Healthy You

Benefits of Some of the Most Popular Herbs and Spices:

- Rosemary and basil are anti-inflammatory

- Cumin, turmeric, and sage fight dementia

- Cayenne, coriander, and cinnamon help to regulate insulin and burn fat

- Lemon grass, nutmeg, bay leaves, and saffron have a calming effect

- Turmeric fights cancer and helps prevent Alzheimer's disease

- Oregano is anti-fungal and antibacterial

- Garlic, mustard seed, and chicory are excellent for the heart

- Basil and thyme help your skin become softer and smoother

- Turmeric, garlic, basil, cinnamon, thyme, saffron, garlic, and ginger boost the immune system

- Coriander, rosemary, cayenne, allspice, and black pepper help banish depression

Recipes From the Kitchen of Margianna

Following are some of my favorite recipes, many in which I have substituted ingredients to be more nutritious or to sidestep my allergies or food intolerances. Unlike Layla, I do not have photos of my recipes; nevertheless, I assure you they are tasty!

Almond-Crusted Wild Salmon Fillets on a Bed of Wilted Greens

1/2 cup chopped almonds
1/4 cup chopped fresh flat-leaf parsley
1 Tbsp. grated organic lemon zest
1/2 tsp. sea salt
1 large egg
2 wild-caught skinless salmon fillets (6-8 oz. each)
2 Tbsp. extra-virgin olive oil, Ghee, or avocado oil
4 cups mixed organic baby greens, spinach, or watercress
Lemon wedges

1. Mix the almonds, parsley, lemon zest, sea salt, and freshly ground black pepper to taste in a wide, shallow bowl.

2. Beat the egg in another wide, shallow bowl.

3. Pat the salmon dry with a paper towel.

4. Dip a salmon fillet in the egg, turning to coat both sides.

5. Transfer the fillet to the bowl with the almond mixture, and press firmly until the almonds adhere. Set aside and repeat with the second fillet.

6. Warm the oil in a large skillet over medium heat. Add the salmon and cook, turning once, until it's opaque in the center, about 5–7 minutes.

7. Arrange 2 cups of greens per plate, and place a cooked salmon fillet on top of the greens.

8. Garnish with lemon wedges and serve immediately.

Mike Geary's Fat-Burning Healthy Chili Recipe

1.5 lbs of a healthy type of ground meat

1 large red pepper, diced

5–6 jalapeno peppers, diced (adjust based on your desired "hotness")

2 large onions, diced

3 tbsp extra-virgin olive oil

2 tbsp pasture-raised butter for added healthy fat and taste

1 large can crushed tomatoes or 5-6 large fresh tomatoes, diced

1 can of kidney beans or black beans

Half a bag of frozen chopped spinach

2 tbsp molasses

3–4 squares of extra dark chocolate (sounds weird, but trust me . . . this adds just a touch of great extra flavor, and a little bit of extra antioxidants)

1 or 2 tbsp of chili powder

1 or 2 tsp of cumin

1 or 2 tbsp of crushed garlic

Add some cayenne pepper to the mix if you like extra hot food

Couple small pinches of sea salt

Add some fresh chopped cilantro while it's cooking

Avocado (for use as a topping after chili is cooked and served)

Grass-fed raw cheese

1. Use a large pot and start with the olive oil, butter, and ground meat cooking.

2. Start adding all of the diced vegetables and other ingredients as you get them ready.

3. If you want to get a little crazy, and increase the nutrition content of this chili even further, you can mix the ground meat you're using with ground grass-fed organ meats since organ meats are nutrient-dense.

4. Once it's all together and cooking in the pot, reduce heat to low and simmer for 40–50 minutes.

5. Top each bowl with freshly diced ripe avocado and sprinkle with shredded cheese.

Shredded Veggies, Beets, Broccoli, or Cauliflower

Easy, nutritious, and delicious recipe that I concocted.

1 package, fresh shredded or "noodled" beets, broccoli, or cauliflower
8 oz package fresh or frozen vegetables (broccoli, cauliflower, carrots, or any you prefer)
1 large onion, chopped
1–2 cloves garlic or 1 tsp ground garlic powder
Salt
Other seasonings as desired

1. Sauté onions and garlic in butter or butter/ghee mixture.

2. Add shredded beets and frozen vegetables, and cook until vegetables are done.

3. Season as preferred with sea salt, black pepper, turmeric, 5-Spices.

4. If you want a sweeter taste, add a little Agave.

For a main dish, add the following to the above recipe:

1 package Quinoa and Brown rice cooked as instructed on the package (I've bought the Quinoa/Brown Rice package at Sam's Club and Sprouts.)
1–2 cups cooked chicken

1. Mix quinoa and brown rice with chicken into shredded beets, broccoli or cauliflower and enjoy as an entrée.

Creamy Corn (bread) Casserole

1/2 cup butter, melted

2 eggs, beaten

1 (8.5 oz) package dry corn bread mix (I substitute a gluten-free mix)

1 (15 oz) can whole kernel corn, drained

1 (14.5 oz) can creamed corn

Add Agave if desired

1 cup sour cream (I substitute goat's milk yogurt because of my cow's milk allergy)

1. Preheat oven to 350° F.

2. Lightly grease a 9x9 inch baking dish or line with parchment paper.

3. In a medium bowl, combine butter, eggs, corn bread mix, whole and creamed corn, and sour cream or yogurt.

4. Spoon mixture into prepared dish.

5. Bake for 45 minutes in preheated oven or until the top is golden brown.

One of my favorites!

Creamy Roasted Avocado

Avocados are a superfood full of fiber, omega-3s, and antioxidants and taste amazing! One nutrition guru reported that eating a slice of avocado with each meal will help to better digest and absorb nutrients from other foods.

2 avocados, halved and pitted

2 tsp lime juice (I didn't have lime juice so I used lemon juice)

1 tsp pureed garlic

1/2 tsp sea salt

2 Tbsp seeds – pumpkin, sesame, or flax

1. Preheat oven to 350° F and place the avocado halves in a greased glass baking dish, flesh-side up.

2. Sprinkle the flesh of avocado with 1/2 tsp of lime or lemon juice.

3. Spread 1/4 tsp of pureed garlic over each half, then sprinkle each with 1/8 tsp of sea salt.

4. Bake in oven for 25 minutes, until tender and creamy.

5. Sprinkle 1/2 Tbsp seeds on top and turn oven to broil and cook for 1–2 minutes until golden brown.

Brain-Boosting Smoothies

"When you eat for your brain, you will think more clearly and efficiently," says Daniel Amen, MD, author of *Unleash the Power of the Female Brain*. The following smoothies from Dr. Amen are packed with foods that help boost blood flow, stabilize blood sugar, and neutralize free radical damage—all important for brain health.

Anti-Inflammatory Smoothie

Inflammation is just as bad for your brain as it is for your body. Chia seeds are high in omega-3 fatty acids, which experts believe are necessary for transmitting signals between brain cells. Blueberries and raspberries are also known for encouraging healthy connections between the cells of the brain.

1/2 cup blueberries

1/2 cup raspberries

1/2 small banana, peeled and frozen

1/4 cup diced pineapple

2 Tbsp chia seeds

3 ice cubes

1/2 cup pomegranate juice

1 serving whey protein powder (vanilla)

1. Combine all the ingredients except the protein powder in a blender, and blend at high speed.
2. Add the protein powder and lightly blend until incorporated.

Banana-Coconut Smoothie

"Coconut is low in natural sugars, high in fiber and manganese, and nature's richest source of medium-chain triglycerides," says Dr. Amen. Medium-chain triglycerides are converted into a stable source of fuel for your brain during periods of low blood sugar and can even help with memory loss.

  1 cup milk (hemp, almond, rice, or organic 1% cow's milk)

  1 frozen banana, slightly thawed

  1 scoop protein powder

  2 Tbsp unsweetened coconut

Combine all ingredients in a blender and blend well.

Almond Smoothie

Almonds are full of dopamine and protein, giving you a "boost of motivation and focus," states Dr. Amen. The ground ginger helps support a robust metabolism, while the cinnamon works to keep your blood sugar steady.

   1 small frozen banana, sliced

   3/4 cup kale, lightly packed, stems removed

   3/4 cup almond milk

   3/4 Tbsp almond butter

   1/8 tsp cinnamon

   1/8 tsp nutmeg

   1/8 tsp ground ginger

Combine all ingredients in a blender and blend until smooth.

Pomegranate-Strawberry Smoothie

Fiber helps regulate blood sugar. And since glucose is your brain's chief source of energy, it's important to keep those levels steady. This low-cal smoothie is full of fiber along with other brain-friendly antioxidants.

1/3 cup pomegranate juice

2 tsp raw honey

3/4 cup frozen unsweetened strawberries

2 Tbsp fat-free plain yogurt

1 Tbsp flaxseed oil

4 ice cubes

1. Whisk pomegranate juice and honey in a small cup to dissolve the honey completely.

2. Combine the strawberries, yogurt, oil, ice cubes, and pomegranate mixture in a blender. Process for 1 to 2 minutes or until thick and smooth.

3. Pour into a glass.

Blueberry Beet Almond Smoothie

Beets are high in fiber, phytonutrients, folate, beta carotene, and natural nitrates that increase blood flow to the brain. (Try this beet smoothie for high blood pressure.)

1/2 cup unsweetened carrot juice

1/2 cup frozen or fresh blueberries

1/2 cup peeled and grated raw beet

1/2 cup unsweetened applesauce

1/2 cup unsalted raw whole almonds

1/2 cup ice cubes

1/2 tsp fresh lime juice

dash of ground ginger

Combine all ingredients in a blender, and blend until smooth and creamy. Serve immediately.

Mango-Avocado Smoothie

Avocados are rich in vitamin E, which has been shown to help reduce the risk of Alzheimer's disease. The spinach offers brain-supporting omega-3s and also helps replenish your iron supply.

1/2 fresh mango

1 cup fresh spinach

1 cup chilled low-fat vanilla soy milk

1/4 avocado

5 tsp agave nectar

Puree all ingredients in a blender until smooth, 1 to 2 minutes. Then, enjoy!

Green Tea and Blueberry Smoothie

Besides containing antioxidants, green tea also has theanine, an amino acid that helps you focus and relax at the same time, according to Dr. Amen. The honey contains all 22 essential amino acids, which provide the building blocks of protein for brain cells.

3 Tbsp water

1 green tea bag

2 tsp raw honey

1-1/2 cups frozen blueberries

1/2 medium banana

3/4 cup calcium-fortified light vanilla soy milk

1. Heat water until steaming hot.

2. Add tea bag and let steep for 3 minutes. Remove tea bag.

3. Stir honey into tea until dissolved. Blend all ingredients (including the tea) on the highest setting until smooth.

Flourless Almond Butter Chocolate Chip Mini Blender Muffins

1 medium ripe banana, peeled

1 large egg

1/2 heaping cup creamy almond butter or peanut butter

3 tablespoons honey (may substitute agave or maple syrup)

1 tablespoon vanilla extract

1/4 teaspoon baking soda

Pinch salt, optional and to taste

Heaping 1/2 cup mini semi-sweet chocolate chips

1. Preheat oven to 400°F. Prepare mini muffin pans by greasing and sprinkling flour in the pans; set aside.

2. Add first 7 ingredients to a blender, through optional salt, and blend on high speed until smooth and creamy, about 1 minute.

3. Add chocolate chips and stir in by hand; don't use the blender because it will pulverize them.

4. Using a tablespoon or small cookie scoop that's been sprayed with cooking spray (helps batter slide off spoon or scoop easily), form rounded 1 tablespoon mounds and place mounds into prepared pans. Each cavity should be filled to a solid 3/4 full.

5. Bake for 8 to 9 minutes, or until the tops are set, springy to the touch, and a toothpick inserted into the center comes out clean with no batter.

6. Allow muffins to cool in pans for about 10 minutes, or until they've firmed up and are cool enough to handle.

Dark Chocolate Avocado Brownies (flourless)

8 ounces melted dark chocolate

2 well-mashed avocados

4 eggs

1 cup of sugar (I substitute agave)

1/2 cup of cocoa powder

1/2 cup of almond meal

1/2 tsp salt

2 tsp vanilla

1. Melt the chocolate.
2. In a medium bowl, whisk together the eggs and sugar (or agave) until very light and doubled in volume.
3. Gradually add in the melted chocolate. Stir in the almond meal, cocoa powder, salt, and vanilla.
4. Blend in the mashed avocado.
5. Pour into a lined or well-greased square baking pan. Bake at 350° for 20–25 minutes.
6. Allow to cool completely before cutting.

Chocolate Avocado Pudding Recipe

(When I served this, none of my friends, including Layla, could identify avocado as an ingredient in the recipe.)

1 medium avocado, ripe

2 Tbsp unsweetened cocoa powder

2 Tbsp honey (maple syrup or agave) – add more to taste if needed

6 Tbsp almond milk or coconut milk

1/2 tsp Vanilla extract

1. Cut open the avocado, discard the pit, and scoop out the avocado. Cut into large chunks and put in the blender.
2. Add cocoa, honey (maple syrup or agave), and milk.
3. Blend, starting on low and then moving to high speed until it is smooth. Refrigerate the pudding and serve cold.

Enjoy plain or with fruit!

Chocolate Nut Delights

1 - 10 oz package Semi-sweet Ghirardelli Chocolate Wafers

1–2 cups chopped pecans

1. Melt chocolate in frying pan.

2. When melted, add pecans.

3. Place in greased muffin tin or spoon onto wax paper and leave to harden.

(Some of my friends said this was the most delicious chocolate dessert they had eaten. . . *Shhh!* Don't divulge how quick and easy it was to make!)

Snacks

Almond Butter

Spread almond butter on natural or non-dairy cheese or banana. Add a "fruit-only" jelly if desired.

Crystallized Low Sugar Ginger Chunks

I soak the ginger in filtered water several times before eating to remove excess sugar.

Apple and Pecan Salad

1. Cut 2–4 apples into small pieces

2. To apples, add the following:

   - Roasted chopped pecans
   - Grapes
   - Dried cranberries
   - Celery
   - Paul Newman's Poppy Seed Dressing

To transform the above salad from a snack food to an entrée, add chopped chicken.

Section Five
~
Odds and Ends

The Odds and Ends section includes internet sites, books, and newsletters that will allow you to continue to learn about anti-aging, nutrition, and supportive lifestyles. Additionally included are tips that I have learned that are helpful in maintaining a healthy lifestyle, taking flattering photographs, saving money, putting an end to junk mail, and more. Enjoy this information and use it to improve your life.

Internet sites, books, newsletters, etc.

DailyOM *(http://www.dailyom.com/)*

DailyOM has beneficial courses and will allow you to choose how much you wish to pay (from $10 to $25) for its courses! These courses give simple step-by-step written instructions in weekly lessons to address specific health and happiness information. Some course titles include:

- Reinventing the Body, Resurrecting the Soul - Dr. Deepak Chopra
- Anti-Aging Face Yoga - Danielle Collins
- Blast Your Brain Fog Away – Dr. Carolyn George & Meeka Anne
- Turn Back the Clock Naturally – Kristen Becker
- Reinventing Happiness – Deepak Chopra & Sonja Lyubomirsky
- 8 Week Whole Body Makeover - Jannine Murray

Great Books on Regenerating Brain Cells

- *BrainSAVE!* by Dr. Titus Chiu, Functional Neurologist. A program to repair and regenerate brain cells: quizzes to determine areas of the brain that need repair, exercises to repair the damage discovered, and lifestyle changes to create new brain cells.

- *The Neurogenesis Diet & Lifestyle: Upgrade Your Brain, Upgrade Your Life* by Brant Cortright, PhD, Clinical Psychologist. "The quality of your brain determines the quality of your life and the quality of your life determines the quality of your brain" and the ways to incorporate changes in your life to support your brain.

- *The Concussion Repair Manual: A Practical Guide to Recovering from Traumatic Brain Injuries* by Dr. Dan Engle. A user's guide with lots of information if you are willing to read a "textbook" type book with medical technology and leading research.

Informative Newsletters – *access and determine those that address your interests.*

- Keith Scott-Mumby, MD: profkeith@alternative-doctor.com
- GreenMedInfo: newsletter@greenmedinfo.com
- Naturecast: news@naturecastproducts.com
- Mark Hyman, MD: drhyman@drhyman.com
- Marc Micozzi, MD: drmarcmicozzi@drmicozzi.com
- Amen Clinics: hello@amenclinics.com

Tips for Simplifying Your Life

Antiperspirants

- There is a great controversy on whether antiperspirants are harmless or harmful because of an article published on the internet several years ago that suggested that they cause cancer. Is it true or false? I don't know.

What I do know is that they contain aluminum, which blocks sweat, and I personally will not take a chance that this metal may be causing negative health issue. (One personally difficult side effect is it causes underarm itching.)

- Natural deodorant products can be found in the grocery stores (if you look closely). The one I like the best is Crystal Body Deodorant Roll-on; it is hypoallergenic, fragrance- and paraben-free, and without harmful aluminum. Many other good quality deodorants are available at health food stores and stores like Sprouts, Whole Foods Market, and Trader Joe's.

Secret of Taking Good Photographs
- If you want to look good and radiant in photographs, dramatize your eyes and face with makeup. Defining your brows and outlining your eyes and mouth highlights your face in photographs.

Prolong the life of skin products and cosmetics
- When a skin cream can no longer be squeezed out of the tube, cut off the top and be amazed at the generous amount of product therein.

- Extend the life of mascara when no longer available from the tube by adding several drops of filtered water to the tube, shake, and continue using many more times.

Shower Caps
- Buy a package of shower caps used by hairdressers at a beauty supply store or other beauty supplier and you will have enough caps to use a new one every couple of weeks for a year. You'll be saving money and avoiding dirt and other harmful things accumulating on or in your cap.

Body Soap

- If sensitive to bar soaps with fragrances or other chemicals, use natural dish soap in the shower or tub. Caution, I do not use any soap on my face (only use makeup removing creams or liquids) and use Ultra Palmolive Soft Touch with Aloe & Citrus or Seventh Generation dish soap to clean my hands and body.

Stop Paper Catalogues (Junk mail)

- https://www.catalogchoice.org

New Font

- A font called *Sans Forgetica* has been scientifically designed to aid people in better remembering information they read. The theory behind this is that when an obstruction (hard-to-read font) gets in the way of reading easily, people remember the content better. http://sansforgetica.rmit/

Germ-Free Program

- Toothbrush: change at least once per month. (I keep a supply purchased inexpensively from a dollar store.)

- Avoid taking your cell phone into the bathroom: studies have shown that the cell phone is then contaminated with harmful germs.

- Avoid using electronic hand dryers: they spread germs, bacteria, etc., and can even spread remains of opioids found on bathroom walls and counters.

Kitchen Dirt

Be sure to take care of the five dirtiest areas:

1. **Kitchen sink:** microbiologist say that there is more E. coli in a kitchen sink than in a toilet after you flush it! Clean daily with antibacterial wipes such as Lysol or Clorox Wipes. (So that's why dogs drink out of the toilet!)

2. **Kitchen sponge:** because the sponge is wet and moist, it soaks up bacteria and many have salmonella growing on them. Microwave wet sponges for 1-2 minutes each day, and then put them into the dishwasher to be cleaned. Use paper towels instead of sponges to clean spills and antibacterial kitchen wipes to clean counters. Replace sponges monthly and inexpensively from a dollar store.

3. **Cutting board:** cutting boards contain more bacteria than toilet seats and, when used to cut poultry and meats, may contain salmonella and other harmful bacteria. Wash the board in hot, soapy water after use and put in the dishwasher or disinfect with bleach (2 tablespoons bleach to 1 gallon of water). Use separate cutting boards for meat/poultry and veggies.

4. **Refrigerator door handle:** opening the door and wiping it with a kitchen sponge invites E. coli, salmonella, and other bacteria to grow on the handle. Wipe every day with disinfecting kitchen wipes.

5. **Kitchen counter:** lots of germs accumulate from chopping veggies, cutting meats, pouring milk, splashes from the sink, and using the kitchen sponge to wipe up spills. Clean counters with disinfecting kitchen wipes and mop up spills with paper towels.

Section Six

~

Recapture Your Youth 8-Week Plan

Week 1
Your Subconscious Beliefs

It is absolutely essential that you have a supportive mindset to reverse aging in the brain and body. Consequently, the first week's focus will be to make sure you have a positive mindset and automatically anticipate success. If this is not innately part of your subconscious mind and you have a negative outlook, it is important that you consistently practice the following program.

Belief System

1. Do you choose to be young? Yes ____ Not now ____

2. What identity have you created for yourself?

   ___ Do you think of yourself as young and vibrant, no matter your age?

   ___ When you get out of bed, are you looking forward to the day?

   ___ Do you have purpose/goals in life for when you retire?

   ___ Are you healthy and energetic?

   ___ Are you happy with your life?

3. How will you change your negative identity?

   a. Afformations. (Noah St. John)_____

   b. Write positive statement at bedtime. (Dr. John Kappas)_____

   c. Speak and think only positive words._____

   d. Say *thank you* many times a day._____

   e. Visualize positive outcomes._____

   f. All of the above._____

Week 2
Your Purpose

Research has proven that having a purpose in life will increase longevity, including for seniors. Older people with a purpose are less likely to have health problems and will more likely enjoy a full, happy life after retirement.

Purpose

1. My purpose is _____.

2. How I will improve someone's life today?

   a. Random Acts of Kindness. Describe: _____.

   b. Offer kind words or encouragement to family or friend. To whom?
   _____.

   c. Hug family and friends. Who and how many?_____
   _____.

   d. Give of my abundant blessings:_____.

   e. The volunteer service for which I will commit weekly:_____
   _____.

   f. Other: _____.

Week 3
Choose Happiness

You are the only person in charge of your happiness! If you don't feel like smiling, fake it 'til you make it! The following practices will help convert unhappiness to happiness.

Choose to be Happy

1. When you have negative thoughts, ask yourself:

    a. Is it true?

    b. Am I projecting the future?

    c. What is true at this moment?

2. Smile!

    a. First thing in the morning, look in the mirror, stand up straight, put your shoulders back and chin up, and smile for 60 seconds.

    b. Smile when you are tense or feeling crummy, such as when you are stuck in traffic or down with a headache.

    c. Consciously smile all day long for at least one week. Fake it until you make it.

3. Laugh

    a. Look in the mirror and fake a laugh (ha, ha, ha) for 60 seconds several times a day. (Tell yourself or a friend a joke.)

4. Hug at least three people each day, or if you do not encounter people to hug, imagine hugging three people, better yet, a handsome man or a beautiful woman.

5. Sing throughout the day!

**Smile and laugh yourself to health and happiness while
you also are giving others a gift of joy!**

Week 4
Repair Your Brain Cells With Diet and Exercise

The focus this week will be on repairing your brain cells and/or stimulating the growth of new ones. The first and most essential activities will be to clean up your diet and start exercising.

Consult your doctor for approval before changing your diet or beginning any exercise program.

Throw out junk foods, including those with sugar and artificial sweeteners. Your diet should consist mainly of fish, beef, poultry, vegetables, and fruit. To satisfy any hunger you have between meals, divide what you would normally eat in three large meals into six smaller meals to keep your blood sugar stable and promote losing weight.

Diet

1. Eliminate sugar, processed and artificial foods, and other foods with chemicals.

2. Eat wild salmon or other wild-caught oily fish at least two times week. (Salmon patties are easy to make from canned, wild salmon and tasty with eggs for breakfast or with veggies for dinner.)

3. Eat four to five servings of vegetables, organic if possible, each day (see recipes herein for salads and for shredded beets, broccoli, or cauliflower).

4. Avocado — eat at least 1 small or ½ medium avocado daily.

5. Add garlic, turmeric, cinnamon, and onions to cooked foods when possible.

6. Snack on:

   - Blueberries, raspberries, and limited dark chocolate daily
   - Natural or fake cheese smothered with almond butter and all-fruit jelly
   - Organic apples, papaya, and grapes

Foods for the Brain

Eat "super" foods daily for brain health.

1. Omega-3 (DHA) foods three times a week — salmon, tuna, halibut, flax and chia seeds, and walnuts

2. Purple, red, and blue grapes

3. Blueberries

4. Strawberries and raspberries

5. Apples

6. Avocados

7. Leafy greens – kale, spinach

8. Broccoli

9. Brussels sprouts

10. Beets

11. Peppers

12. Tomatoes

13. Swiss cheese

14. Olive oil

15. Almond butter

16. Ghee

Physical Exercise

Add physical exercise to your program to increase your blood and lymphatic circulation, tone and build muscles and, importantly, rebuild or create new brain cells.

1. My best aerobic and strength building exercise is _____ _____ and I commit to doing it ____ times a week for ____ minutes. (walking, yoga, dancing, swimming, strength training/weight lifting)

    or

    Walk or perform other aerobic exercise for at least 30 minutes three times a week and resistance exercises for at least 15 minutes three times a week.

2. Each morning, perform the five-minute **Eden Daily Energy Routine**, https://edenenergymedicine.com/donnas-daily-energy-routine/, to energize the body and brain.

3. If you experience "senior moments" or other memory problems, carry out the exercises in Dr. Titus Chiu's book, ***BrainSAVE!,*** https://www.amazon. com/s?k=brain+save+book&crid=1LY8HL06MGLFG&sprefix=Brain+Save %2Caps%2C164&ref=nb_sb_ss_i_1_10

Week 5
Brain Cell Regeneration - Mental Stimulation and Brain Function Supplements

The focus this week will be on continuing to repair your brain cells and/or stimulate the growth of new ones.

Mental Stimulation

1. Reduce TV time

2. Increase brain stimulants

   a. Read

   b. Write - journal, e-mails, texts, stories, poems, articles

   c. Research interesting topics on the internet

   d. Play mental/brain games

   e. Discuss serious issues with family and friends

   f. Participate in hobbies

      • Crafts – knitting, crocheting, etc.

      • Art

g.   Learn a foreign language or musical instrument

3.   Organize your life, home, and business

Supplements

There are many supplements to enhance brain function; however, it is best to eat and exercise for your brain first and then find a functional health doctor to determine what supplements your brain needs to function optimally.

> **Consult your doctor for approval before taking supplements—some will interfere with prescription drugs.**

General Brain and Body Health Supplements:

Check your Vitamin D and Magnesium levels and consult your doctor about supplementing if deficient. It is reported that the majority of Americans are deficient in these nutrients.

Brain Repair:

- Vitamin D3 — reduces risks of dementia

- Magnesium L-threonate – crosses blood brain barrier to stabilize unstable brain cells

- Liposomal glutathione – the brain's master anti-oxidant

- Ginkgo Biloba – improves circulation to brain cells and protects the brain from stress-induced cell death

- Curcumin – natural anti-inflammatory

Dr. Mary Newport's Recommendation for Brain Repair:

Mix 16 ounces of MCT oil with 12 ounces of coconut oil and store at room temperature so it will stay liquid. The level of ketones in coconut oil increases slowly and peaks from 3 to 7 hours while MCT oil peaks after 90 minutes, so you get the benefit of both immediate and long-term ketones by adding them together. Take a half teaspoon to one teaspoon, especially when introducing MCT oil to your diet. Increase over two or three days and work up to 4-6 tablespoons a day (or even more if tolerated, divided over two to four meals.)

Other Ways to Use MCT Oil and Coconut Oil:

1. Mix coconut oil or MCT oil with almond butter that is freshly ground.

2. Soften butter (preferably organic) or Ghee at room temperature and mix with coconut oil or MCT oil in an equal amount.

3. Cook with coconut oil but at not more than 350 degrees because high heat will alter the fat, destroying the ketones.

4. Add 1 teaspoon to 1 tablespoon of MCT in coffee—it is tasteless.

5. Make salad dressings from coconut or MCT oil or add either to existing salad dressings.

6. Add coconut or MCT oil to smoothies.

Week 6
Spiritual Connection, Sleep, and Voice

Spiritual participation

1. Spiritual group and activity?

2. Spiritual practice:

    a. Meditation practice begun _____

    b. Volunteering _____

3. Helping Others:

    a. Smiling _____

    b. Words of Encouragement _____

    c. Donations _____

Sleep for brain health

1. Sleep 8 hours a night _____

Youthful, Vibrant Voice

1. Sing familiar songs loudly and clearly for 10 minutes daily _____

2. Sing scales, high and low, for 5 minutes daily_____

3. Gargle with warm water for 60 seconds twice daily_____

4. Talk with conviction daily to others or yourself _____

Week 7
Look Young

Determine how you want to look and how much effort you are willing to devote to your look.

Skin and Makeup

1. Determine your representational type.
   I am: Visual____Auditory____Kinesthetic____.

2. Perform "dry brushing" and then apply crepe-defying oils or creams before bathing or showering.

3. Research skin creams for the best one for your skin type that does not have toxic ingredients — buy organic.

4. No soap on the face (unless naturally extremely oily) — apply makeup remover creams or lotions to your face for removing makeup and for skin health.

5. After applying face cream, exercise your face for 5-10 minutes each morning.

6. Apply makeup using techniques described herein or on makeup sites.

7. Smile to hide imperfections and to make your face more beautiful.

Hair

1. Incorporate a lifestyle that promotes healthy hair: healthy diet, exercise, adequate sleep, elimination of stress.

2. Purchase and use non-toxic hair products.

3. For shine and frizz reduction, apply organic, natural almond oil to hair.

4. If your hair is thinning, investigate supplements such as fish oil, B-complex, and Life Code's Stem Cell or Telomax.

5. Have fun virtually trying on hundreds of hairstyles and discover information to enhance your look at **https://www.thehairstyler.com/face-shape-quiz.** Go to **https://www.thehairstyler.com/** or **https://www.thehairstyler.com/virtual-hairstyler**.

Week 8
Your Look Continued:
Clothing Styles, Colors, and Bargains

1. Determine your clothing style. My dominant style is_____.

2. I'm warm or cool on the color scale?_____ and _____season.

3. My body type is: Apple____Pear____Rectangular____Hourglass ___

4. Shopping guidelines in order :

    a. Look for size

    b. Look for my colors

    c. Look for style

    d. Look for bargains!

Celebrate the new you!!!

Section Seven
~
Resource Section

Choose to be Young

Holman, Steve, and Beck Homan, eds. n.d., Iron Man Magazine. https://www.ironmanmagazine.com/.

Doidge, Norman. 2007. *The Brain That Changes Itself: Stories of Personal Triumph from the Frontiers of Brain Science*. New York: Penguin Books.

As You Thinketh

"Re-Programming Your Subconscious Mind: A New Script for Health and Relationships With Dr. Bruce Lipton." Face the Current, October 7, 2018. https://facethecurrent.com/bruce-lipton-3/. *Note:* Dr. Bruce Lipton can also be found at https://www.brucelipton.com

St. John, Noah. *Book of Afformations: Discovering the Missing Piece to Abundant Health, Wealth, Love, and Happiness*. Carlsbad: Hay House, 2013.

Kappas, John G. *Success Is Not an Accident: The Mental Bank Concept*. Van Nuys, Calif.: Panorama Publishing Co., 1987.

"Oprah Winfrey Quotes to Charge Your Day with Gratitude." Goalcast, July 27, 2017. https://www.goalcast.com/2017/07/27/7-oprah-winfrey-quotes-to-charge-your-day-with-gratitude/.

Sukyo Mahikari. *Gratitude*. Takayama City: Sukyo Mahikari, 2003.

Aimee Copeland: The Official Site, n.d. https://aimeecopeland.com/.

Wright, Carolanne. "Research Says Gratitude Can Reverse Aging, Stress and Ill Health." NaturalNews.com, October 17, 2014. http://www.naturalnews.com/047287_gratitude_reverse_aging_stress.html.

Chopra, Deepak. "Cultivate the Healing Power of Gratitude." The Chopra Center, October 30, 2017. http://www.chopra.com/ccl/cultivate-the-healing-power-of-gratitude.

"The New Science of Gratitude." Science of Gratitude, n.d. http://gratitudepower.net/science.htm.

Purpose in Life

Miller, Jen A., n.d. http://jenamiller.com/.

Bennett, David A., Julie A. Schneider, Aron S. Buchman, Lisa L. Barnes, Patricia A. Boyle, and Robert S. Wilson. "Overview and Findings from the Rush Memory and Aging Project." *Current Alzheimer Research.* 9, no. 6 (2012): 646–63. https://doi.org/10.2174/156720512801322663.

Rebok, George W. "The Baltimore Experience Corps Study." Rep. *The Baltimore Experience Corps Study.* Johns Hopkins University, September 19, 2013. https://clinicaltrials.gov/ct2/show/NCT00380562.

Amen, Daniel G. *Use Your Brain to Change Your Age: Secrets to Look, Feel, and Think Younger Every Day.* New York: Three Rivers Press, 2012.

Ni, Maoshing. *Secrets of Longevity: Hundreds of Ways to Live to Be 100.* San Francisco: Chronicle, 2006.

"A Quote by Virginia Satir." Goodreads, n.d. https://www.goodreads.com/quotes/98328-we-need-4-hugs-a-day-for-survival-we-need.

Happiness is Your Choice

Rose, Mark. *Heaven on Earth Book 1.* Manhattan, Kan.: The Claflin Media Group, 2014.

Spector, Nicole. "Smiling Can Trick Your Brain into Happiness - and Boost Your Health." NBCNews.com. NBCUniversal News Group, November 28, 2017. https://www.nbcnews.com/better/health/smiling-can-trick-your-brain-happiness-boost-your-health-ncna822591.

Sarlin, Peggy, and David Perlmutter. Awakening from Alzheimer's: The Event. Other. *Awakening from Alzheimer's*. Online Publishing & Marketing LLC, 2016.

Ekman, Paul. *Non-Verbal Messages: Cracking the Code: My Life's Pursuit*. San Francisco: Paul Ekman Group, 2016.

O'Connor, Joseph, and John Seymour. *Introducing NLP: Psychological Skills for Understanding and Influencing People*. London: Thorsons, 1990.

It's All in Your Head — Regenerate Your Brain

Amen, Daniel G. *Use Your Brain to Change Your Age: Secrets to Look, Feel, and Think Younger Every Day*. New York: Three Rivers Press, 2012.

"Biohacking Your Brain's Health from Coursera." Emory University, n.d. https://www.class-central.com/course/coursera-biohacking-your-brain-s-health-11544.

Cortright, Brant. *The Neurogenesis Diet and Lifestyle: Upgrade Your Brain, Upgrade Your Life*. Mill Valley, Calif: Psyche Media, 2015.

"Facts and Figures." Alzheimer's Association. Alzheimer's Association, n.d. https://www.alz.org/alzheimers-dementia/facts-figures.

Fernandez, Alvaro, Elkhonon Goldberg, and Pascale Michelon. *The Sharpbrains Guide to Brain Fitness: How to Optimize Brain Health and Performance at Any Age*. Lexington: Sharpbrains, Inc., 2013.

Grossman, David. "We Can Prevent Dementia." Karolinska University Hospital, May 4, 2017. https://www.karolinska.se/en/karolinska-university-hospital/news/2017/05/miia-kivipelto/.

Lugavere, Max, and Paul Grewal. *Genius Foods: Become Smarter, Happier, and More Productive While Protecting Your Brain for Life*. New York: Harper Wave, 2018.

Sarlin, Peggy, and Dale Bredesen. "Awakening from Alzheimer's," Episode Transcripts. Online Publishing & Marketing, LLC, 2016

Diet

Sarlin, Peggy, and David Perlmutter. Awakening from Alzheimer's: The Event. Other. *Awakening from Alzheimer's*. Online Publishing & Marketing LLC, 2016.

Amen, Daniel G. *Use Your Brain to Change Your Age: Secrets to Look, Feel, and Think Younger Every Day*. New York: Three Rivers Press, 2012.

Cortright, Brant. *The Neurogenesis Diet and Lifestyle: Upgrade Your Brain, Upgrade Your Life*. Mill Valley, Calif: Psyche Media, 2015.

"Broccoli." GreenMedInfo | Blog Entry, July 25, 2015. http://www.greenmedinfo.com/substance/broccoli.

Zinczenko, David. "Eat This, Not That! No-Diet Weight Loss, Nutrition Tips and More." Eat This Not That, n.d. https://www.eatthis.com/.

Lalanne, Jack. "Feats." Jack Lalanne, n.d. http://jacklalanne.com/feats/.

Exercise

Silver Sneakers, https://www.silversneakers.com/

Dr. Barbara Bergin, n.d. https://drbarbarabergin.com/.

Spirduso, Waneen Wyrick., Leonard W. Poon, and Wojtek J. Chodzko-Zajko. *Exercise and Its Mediating Effects on Cognition*. Champaign, Ill: Human Kinetics, 2008.

Castanet, Craig. Non Surgical Disc Decompression Therapy Decatur GA - Backstrong Non-Surgical Rehab Clinic. Backstrong.net, n.d. https://backstrong.net/.

"7 Symptoms of Sarcopenia." Healthy Info Daily, July 31, 2018. https://healthyinfodaily.com/7-symptoms-of-sarcopenia/.

"List of Weight Training Exercises." Wikipedia. Wikimedia Foundation, December 10, 2018. https://en.wikipedia.org/wiki/List_of_weight_training_exercises.

"Donna's Daily Energy Routine." edenenergymedicine.com, n.d. https://edenenergymedicine.com/donnas-daily-energy-routine/.

Chiu, Titus. *BrainSAVE: the 6-Week Plan to Heal Your Brain from Concussion, Brain Injuries & Trauma without Drugs or Surgery*. Berkeley: The Modern Brain, 2018.

"Posture Exercises: 12 Exercises to Improve Your Posture." Healthline, n.d. https://www.healthline.com/health/posture-exercises#child's-pose-.

"5 Essential Fitness Rules for Older Adults." SilverSneakers, March 1, 2018. https://www.silversneakers.com/blog/5-essential-fitness-rules-older-adults/.

"Victoria Yunsoo Shin, MD" Torrance Memorial Medical Center, n.d. https://www.torrancememorial.org/Find_a_Doctor/Physician_Search/S/Victoria_Yunsoo_Shin_M_D_.aspx.

"Dr. David Kruse." MedFit Network, n.d. https://medfitnetwork.org/about/our-team/dr-david-kruse/.

"SilverSneakers Yoga." SilverSneakers, n.d. https://www.silversneakers.com/class/yoga.

"Strength Exercises for Seniors: Everything You Need to Know." SilverSneakers, July 19, 2018. https://www.silversneakers.com/blog/strength-training-for-seniors/.

"Stretch, Yoga and Tai Chi Videos." Collage Video, n.d. https://www.collagevideo.com/collections/stretch-yogo-and-tai-chi-videos.

"The 28 Day Yoga for Beginners Program." DOYOUYOGA.COM, n.d. https://www.doyouyoga.com/programs/the-yoga-for-beginners-starter-kit/.

Burnell, Anne Pringle. "10 Daily Posture Exercises for Seniors Video." YouTube, March 16, 2011. https://www.youtube.com/watch?v=WJspJaFL_l8&has_verified=1 and.

"Free Exercises For Seniors And The Elderly." Eldergym®, n.d. https://eldergym.com/exercises/.

"5 Essential Fitness Rules for Older Adults." SilverSneakers, March 1, 2018. https://www.silversneakers.com/blog/5-essential-fitness-rules-older-adults/.

Supplements

Geda, Y. E., H. M. Topazian, R. A. Lewis, R. O. Roberts, D. S. Knopman, V. S. Pankratz, T. J. H. Christianson, et al. "Engaging in Cognitive Activities, Aging, and Mild Cognitive Impairment: A Population-Based Study." *Journal of Neuropsychiatry* 23, no. 2 (April 2011): 149–54. https://doi.org/10.1176/appi.neuropsych.23.2.149.

"Going Outside—Even in the Cold—Improves Memory, Attention." University of Michigan, December 16, 2008. https://news.umich.edu/going-outsideeven-in-the-coldimproves-memory-attention/.

Cooper, Simon B., Stephan Bandelow, Maria L. Nute, Karah J. Dring, Rebecca L. Stannard, John G. Morris, and Mary E. Nevill. "Sprint-Based Exercise and Cognitive Function in Adolescents." *Preventive Medicine Reports* 4 (December 2016): 155–61. https://doi.org/10.1016/j.pmedr.2016.06.004.

Stathokostas, Liza. "Can Weight Training Boost the Aging Brain?" Western University, n.d. https://www.uwo.ca/ccaa/research/stories/weights_brain.html.

Cortright, Brant. *The Neurogenesis Diet and Lifestyle: Upgrade Your Brain, Upgrade Your Life*. Mill Valley, Calif: Psyche Media, 2015.

Sarlin, Peggy, and Mary Newport. Awakening from Alzheimer's: The Event. Other. *Awakening from Alzheimer's*. Online Publishing & Marketing LLC, 2016.

"Dr. Mary Newport, Alzheimer's Disease: What If There Was A Cure?" Coconut Ketones, n.d. https://coconutketones.com/.

Chiu, Titus. *BrainSAVE: the 6-Week Plan to Heal Your Brain from Concussion, Brain Injuries & Trauma without Drugs or Surgery*. Berkeley: The Modern Brain, 2018.

Engle, Dan. *The Concussion Repair Manual: a Practical Guide to Recovering from Traumatic Brain Injuries*. Las Vegas: Lifestyle Entrepreneurs Press, 2017.

Spiritual

Pargament, Kenneth I., and Harold Koenig. *The Psychology of Religion and Coping: Theory, Research, Practice*. New York: Guilford Press, 1997.

Newberg, Andrew B., and Mark Robert Waldman. *How God Changes Your Brain: Breakthrough Findings from a Leading Neuroscientist*. New York: Ballantine Books, 2010.

Chopra, Deepak. *The Soul of Healing Meditations: a Simple Approach to Growing Younger*. CD. Rasa Music, n.d. (Can be found on Amazon.com as mp3, CD, or streaming.)

"Guided Healing Meditation." Guided Healing Meditation with Patrick from Samarpan Foundation, Goa, India. Biogetica, n.d. https://www.biogetica.com/patrick-meditation.mp3.

"Guided Secular Healing Meditations." Biogetica, n.d. http://www.biogetica.com/guided-meditations.php.

Scott-Mumby, Keith. "The Power Of Love, Gratitude and Forgiveness." Love, Gratitude and Forgiveness Multi-media Sensory Stimulation, n.d. http://www.advancedmindstrategies.com/.

Sukyo Mahikari. "Sukyo Mahikari North America." Sukyo Mahikari North America - Light Energy, n.d. http://www.sukyomahikari.org/.

Fernandez-Carriba, Samuel. YouTube, July 10, 2018. https://www.youtube.com/watch?v=mbXxo_oZqsY.

Sleep

Amen, Daniel G. *Use Your Brain to Change Your Age: Secrets to Look, Feel, and Think Younger Every Day*. New York: Three Rivers Press, 2012.

Wolfe, David. *Longevity Now*. Berkeley: North Atlantic Books, 2013.

"What Happens In the Brain During Sleep?" *Scientific American Mind* 26, no. 5 (September 2015): 70–70. https://doi.org/10.1038/scientificamericanmind0915-70a.

"Brain Basics: Understanding Sleep." National Institute of Neurological Disorders and Stroke. U.S. Department of Health and Human Services, n.d. https://www.ninds.nih.gov/Disorders/Patient-Caregiver-Education/Understanding-Sleep#8.

Voice

The Body ODD. "The Wavery, Shaky 'Old Person's Voice,' Explained." NBCNews. com. NBCUniversal News Group, January 25, 2013. https://www.nbcnews. com/healthmain/wavery-shaky-old-persons-voice-explained-1C8119298.

Awaken Your Youth — Wrinkles Be Gone

O'Connor, Joseph, and John Seymour. *Introducing NLP: Psychological Skills for Understanding and Influencing People.* London: Thorsons, 1990.

Langston, Margianna. *Unleash the Thin Within: The Spirit, Mind, and Body Solution to Permanent Weight Control.* Atlanta: HBS Strategies, LLC, 2013.

Harlan, Timothy S. *Its Heartly Fare: a Food Book That Makes Sense of Fat, Cholesterol, and Salt.* Atlanta: Pritchett & Hull, 2005.

"Tone & Firm Your Face With Facial Exercises By Happy Face Yoga." Happy Face Yoga, n.d. https://www.happyfaceyoga.com/.

Nadeau, Marie Véronique. *The Yoga Facelift: the All-Natural, Do-It-Yourself Program for Looking Younger and Feeling Better.* San Francisco: Comari Press, 2007 (An updated edition of this book is available.)

Maggio, Carole. *Carole Maggio Facercise.* New York: Berkley Publishing Group, 2002.

Hagen, Annelise. *The Yoga Face: Eliminate Wrinkles with the Ultimate Natural Facelift.* New York: Penguin Group, 2007.

"Dry Brushing Technique." Natural Health Techniques, n.d. https://natural healthtechniques.com/healingtechniquesdry_brushing_technique/.

Manning, Margaret. "*14 Exclusive Makeup Tips for Older Women from a Professional Makeup Artist.*" Sixty and Me, 2017. http://sixtyandme.com/14-exclusive-makeup-tips-for-older-women-from-a-professional-makeup-artist/.

Recommended Products:

"Bell Virtu Organic Nourishing Eye Serum" https://www.amazon.com/gp/product/B00KGJVVDK/ref=oh_aui_detailpage_o04_s00?ie=UTF8&psc=1

"theCream," https://www.thecream.com/

"Asterwood Naturals Matrixyl 3000, Argireline Vitamin C," https://www.amazon.com/

FineVine "Organic Almond Oil," https://www.amazon.com/

Advanced Clinicals' "Green Coffee Bean Oil," "Thermo-Firming Cream," and "Genes Vitamin E Crème, Swiss Collagen Complex for Dry and Sensitive Skin," https://www.amazon.com/

Shinier, Thicker, Healthier Hair

Sears, Al. "*Can McDonald's French Fries Cure Baldness*?" Al Sears, MD, n.d. https://alsearsmd.com/2018/10/can-mcdonalds-french-fries-cure-baldness/.

"*Health and Fitness News, Recipes, Natural Remedies.*" Dr. Axe, n.d. https://draxe.com/. (Search for "supplements to encourage hair health")

"*The Complete List – 15 Harmful Shampoo Ingredients to Avoid.*" Nutrafol, April 16, 2018. https://blog.nutrafol.com/2018/04/16/15-shampoo-ingredients-to-avoid/.

"*Dr Mercola Interviews Dr Villeponteau the Formulator of Stem Cell 100.*" Life Code RSS, n.d. https://www.lifecoderx.com/.

Hair Styles: https://www.thehairstyler.com/face-shape-quiz; https://www.the hairstyler.com/ https://www.thehairstyler.com/virtual-hairstyler

Look Your Best — Clothes to Enhance Your Appearance

Clothes Styles: https://www.proprofs.com/quiz-school/story.php?title=whats-your-personal-fashion-style

Richmond, JoAnne. *Reinvent Yourself with Color Me Beautiful: Four Seasons of Color, Makeup, and Style.* Lanham: Taylor Trade Publishing, 2008.

Recipes

"*Chocolate Lovers Society.*" Facebook. https://www.facebook.com/ (Layla's Facebook group)

Odds & Ends

Courses, DailyOM, http://www.dailyom.com/

Great Books on Regenerating Brain Cells:

- Chiu, Titus. *BrainSAVE: The 6-Week Plan to Heal Your Brain from Concussions, Brain Injuries & Trauma without Drugs or Surgery.* The Modern Brain: Berkeley, 2018.

- Cortright, Brant. *The Neurogenesis Diet & Lifestyle, Upgrade Your Brain, Upgrade Your Life.* Psyche Media: Mill Valley, Calif., 2015

- Engle, Dan. *The Concussion Repair Manual.* Lifestyle Entrepreneurs Press: Las Vegas, 2017

Informative Newsletters:

- Keith Scott-Mumby, MD: profkeith@alternative-doctor.com

- GreenMedInfo: newsletter@greenmedinfo.com

- Naturecast: news@naturecastproducts.com

- Mark Hyman, MD: drhyman@drhyman.com

- Marc Micozzi, MD: drmarcmicozzi@drmicozzi.com

- Amen Clinics: hello@amenclinics.com

Stop Paper Catalogues (Junk mail): https://www.catalogchoice.org

New Font: http://sansforgetica.rmit/

Acknowledgements

I am deeply grateful to the many people who have inspired, helped and supported me, including my family and friends. I am also extremely grateful to those that added their expertise to the book's content or allowed me to use their stories, including:

Samuel Fernandez Carriba, PhD, Senior Psychologist, Clinical Assessment and Diagnosis, and Assistant Professor, Department of Pediatrics at Emory University School of Medicine

Craig Castanet, D.C., CEDIR, CFMP, Backstrong Non-Surgical Rehab Clinic, Decompression Therapy, Decatur, GA

Goetz Eaton (my brother-in-law), Judge, Anderson Municipal Court

Layla Lusty, Gourmet Cook (and loving and compassionate friend)

Lee Hong Tan

Supportive friends and book contributors:

Joanne Mitchell

Lynda Ellis

Sue May Goh

Annette Ashizawa (now deceased)

Joan Ouillen

Maricelo Runz

ACKNOWLEDGEMENTS

Production Assistance:

Marcy Pusey, Writing & Publishing Coach, Self-Publishing School

Kim Carr, Editor & Formatter, On The Mark Editorial Services

Alek J., Cover Designer, UpWork

Brandon Reece, Photographer

About the Author

Ms. Langston is a certified Neuro-Linguistic Professional with the Robbins Research Institute, a former Nutritional Consultant in a medical practice, and an Advanced-level member of Sukyo Mahikari, a spiritual development organization. She is a self-described crusader with a quest for learning and for helping others find health, happiness, and peace of mind.

Ms. Langston has two Bachelor of Science degrees, one from Florida State University, where she majored in Marketing/Business; and another from the now-closed International University of Nutrition Education, with a major in Nutrition and Preventive Health. Additionally, she has completed all coursework for a dual MS/PhD in nutrition, studied with prominent doctors in the nutrition and alternative medicine fields, including Nobel Prize winner, the late Linus Paulding.

www.ingramcontent.com/pod-product-compliance
Lightning Source LLC
Chambersburg PA
CBHW081414270326
41931CB00015B/3277